The Montessori Way

A PRACTICAL GUIDE TO HELP THE CHILD WITH AUTISM SPECTRUM DISORDER (ASD) LEARN USING MONTESSORI INSPIRATION

Rachel Peachey

Sterling Family Production
LEXINGTON, KENTUCKY

Copyright © 2017 by Sterling Family Production

All rights reserved. No part of this publication may be reproduced, distributed or transmitted in any form or by any means, including photocopying, recording, or other electronic or mechanical methods, without the prior written permission of the publisher, except in the case of brief quotations embodied in critical reviews and certain other noncommercial uses permitted by copyright law. For permission requests, write to the publisher, addressed "Attention: Permissions Coordinator," at the address below.

Sterling Family Production
www.sterlingproduction.com
ashleyandmitch@sterlingproduction.com

Autism, The Montessori Way: A Practical Guide to Help the Child with Autism Spectrum Disorder (ASD) Learn Using Montessori Inspiration
Rachel Peachey
ISBN: 978-1974023622
SBN-10: 1974023621

Contents

Introduction 7

A Brief History of Montessori 11

An Overview of Autism.. 17
    Prevalence.. 18
    Diagnosis 18
    ASD Symptoms 19
    Treatment 20
    Strengths of Individuals with ASD 21
    ASD and Other Disorders 22

Early Intervention Using Montessori.................... 27
    The Absorbent Mind 28
    Floortime and Montessori... 29
    Applied Behavior Analysis and Montessori.............. 31
    Montessori Early Intervention Activities for ASD ... 39

Montessori Sensorial   Experiences and Autism 47
    Benefits of Sensorial Activities 48
    Montessori Sensorial Activities 50

Following the Child and Autism 61
    Why is Following the Child Important 62

Guidelines for Following Your Child with ASD 67

Managing Choice and Freedom 77
Freedom and Choice in the Montessori Method 78
Guiding Towards Using Freedom and Choice Responsibly 80

Grace and Courtesy Lessons and Children with ASD 87
Examples of Lessons in Grace and Courtesy 88

Understanding and Responding to Triggers for Children with ASD 95
Understanding Triggers 96
Avoiding and Coping with Triggers 101
The Montessori Environment and Curriculum and Triggers 103
Responding to Outbursts the Montessori Way 107

Conclusion 113

More Titles by Rachel Peachey 115

More Titles by the Producers, A. M. Sterling ... 116

Resources 117

References	117
About the Author	123
About the Publisher	125

To my ever-supportive husband and energizing children.

"Everyone in the world ought to do the things for which he is specially adapted. It is the part of wisdom to recognize what each one of us is best fitted for, and it is the part of education to perfect and utilize such predispositions. Because education can direct and aid nature but can never transform her."
- DR. MARIA MONTESSORI

CHAPTER ONE

Introduction

There's a shift that happens in your brain and life when you learn about Montessori. I often reflect on how different my parenting would have been had I not been introduced to Montessori about a year before I had my first child. Reading Montessori's work and studying the curriculum albums led me to have a completely different understanding of children. Suddenly, children's behavior has greater meaning and purpose. Running through the house in their underwear because they don't want help getting their clothes on is a request for independence and an obsession with pouring water is all about developing motor control. Their struggles and outbursts become windows showing their needs, wants and goals.

If you're a parent of a child with ASD you have been down this road of trying to understand your child. Whether you noticed differences in your child's behavior from an early age, or detected it later, your journey has likely been one of wondering, worrying and trying to understand your child. With a greater understanding of the Montessori method and autism, it is my hope that, you too will have this shift in perspective that I experienced. While it doesn't answer all the questions or solve every single problem you may encounter, the philosophy provides a basis of beliefs and ideas that gives hope and lights a path.

Awareness and understanding of autism spectrum disorder (ASD) has grown greatly over the past fifty years. Better diagnostic services are available and more people are using them. As a result, many more parents and educators are seeking the best educational opportunities for children who are on the spectrum. One popular choice has been the Montessori method.

Because the Montessori method was developed by Dr. Maria Montessori who achieved impressive results in children with special needs in the early 1900s, many hope that her method will help their children learn. There are many positive aspects about the method that make it ideal for working with children with ASD. The method promotes following the child, moving at the child's pace and the use of hands-on and sensory experiences for learning. These, among other aspects of the method, have created a buzz, making many parents wonder if it's the best option for their child with ASD.

Whether you're a parent or an educator, this book was designed to help you learn about both autism and the Montessori method. This book is aimed at helping parents and teachers understand how the Montessori method can be most helpful for children with ASD, and how to respond to typical struggles children with autism have using the method.

There are many ways to incorporate the Montessori method into your child's life. You may decide to homeschool, or place your child in a Montessori school, or perhaps you'll decide to send your child to a traditional school, but use Montessori principles at home. There is no one right or wrong way to do it. Each child is different and will have unique needs. Parents and educators need to work together to find the best combination of activities and therapies for the child.

Whatever you decide, incorporating Montessori into your and your child's life is a wonderful way to approach learning. With an understanding of the basic principles of Montessori and some of the areas where it can most aid your child with autism, you'll start on your journey in learning with a fresh perspective. For many, Montessori's philosophy has greatly changed the way they parent, teach or even view children. This is especially true for children with autism, who require even greater understanding from those who care for them.

Whether you are just beginning to learn about autism and Montessori, or you're already familiar with them, I hope you will find this book helpful on your journey.

CHAPTER TWO

A Brief History of Montessori

Dr. Maria Montessori is the revolutionary woman who developed the popular, world-renowned Montessori method. Although she developed the method over a century ago, her observations and recommendations for education are still relevant and even progressive by today's standards. Montessori's work is particularly relevant to the youngest of children and those with special developmental needs.

Starting out as a doctor trained in Italy, her native home, Montessori shifted her focus to psychology after graduating from medical school in 1896. Fundamental to the development of her method was Montessori's participation in a research program at the psychiatric clinic of the University of Rome in 1897. This experience led her to study two of her major influencers, Jean Marc Gaspard Itard and Edouard Seguin.

She became intrigued by the children at the asylums she visited as a part of her research. It was here that she noticed the lack of stimulation and resources provided to children in these institutions. Slowly, Montessori gained recognition for her new ideas and the work she was doing. This resulted in Montessori's appointment, along with Guisseppe Montesano, as co-director of a new institution called the Orthophrenic School. At this school, children with many kinds of disorders were taught by Montessori. She worked endlessly, teaching and trying learning materials created by Itard and Seguin all day and then writing up her notes and observations at night. She quickly found that the children were capable of much more than anyone had believed possible. Stimulation and access to the right guidance and materials were all the children needed.

Montessori then went on to work with developmentally normal, poor children in a ghetto of Rome. A group of investors hired Montessori to look after children who had free-reign of a new building where factory workers lived. Hoping she could contain the mayhem, the investors essentially asked her to babysit the children. However, Montessori saw it as a golden opportunity to continue practicing her ideas in education. It was here that she developed the meat of the Montessori method. She called the project "Casa dei Bambini." It was here, through careful observation of the children and employment of methods she had previously used in the Orthophrenic School, that she began developing her teaching style.

Montessori also added to the learning materials she had used previously, creating materials such as beads for counting, wooden letters, specially designed blocks and many, many others.

Her perspectives and ideas for working with both developmentally different and poor children were quite surprising at the time. Few other doctors or psychologists had taken an interest in these groups of children. In a time where education typically began at around age 7 for those who were lucky enough to be sent to school, younger children and the marginalized for were almost completely ignored. Montessori changed the way these children were viewed and exposed the potential they truly had.

The philosophy and methodology Montessori created produces amazing results both for developmentally normal and special needs children. Some of the main differences that Montessori offers from traditional schooling methods include:

- No external rewards are used.

- Children learn by manipulating objects and benefit from learning concrete concepts first, and then moving towards abstract concepts.
- Real-life objects are preferred to toys.
- Multi-aged classrooms encourage interaction between younger and older children and offer many benefits as a result.
- The role of the teacher is that of a guide.
- Children are allowed freedom of movement.
- It is believed that children are naturally interested in mastering certain activities and topics when provided with the appropriate guidance, materials and opportunities.
- For a child to learn and discover to her full potential, the teacher must "follow" her. Children show in their actions and interests what they want to learn. It is the teacher's job to cultivate and develop the child's abilities based on her interests.
- Children can learn at their own pace.
- Children are given time to work individually without interruption.
- Children are not empty vessels to be filled, but complete beings who only require freedom, guidance and the opportunity to discover the world around them.
- Young children learn by imitation.
- Subject areas like practical life, social skills and sensory learning are included in the curriculum.

Montessori's methods quickly became popular and schools around the world began practicing Montessori style education. Today, Montessori is very popular in schools, with homeschoolers and with both developmentally normal and special needs students. The full method is a combination of curriculum lessons which Montessori created in great detail, for children ages 0-12. There are middle school and high school Montessori programs, however the curriculum for these levels is a bit less structured. In addition to curriculum guides, Montessori wrote many books and papers about childhood development, the role she believed education played in the world.

Montessori's methods can be easily adapted to each student. Because each student moves at their own pace, and the teacher follows the student's interests and needs, students receive more individualized attention than what is traditionally allowed. This, along with a focus on using concrete materials and developing the senses are some of the features that most make Montessori appropriate for use with children who have special needs, including children with ASD.

As you explore the world of Montessori, you'll find that there are many different accreditation institutions schools and curriculums reference. There isn't one body that oversees Montessori education, so if you're looking for a school or curriculum, it's best to visit and ask lots of questions to find out if it's what you're looking for. As you become more familiar with the method, try reading some of Montessori's original writings! Even though much of her work was written long ago, it's still relevant today.

Throughout this book, some of the most important ways that Montessori is helpful for children with autism spectrum disorders will be outlined. In addition, recommended modifications and special considerations for ASD children are also discussed.

"I felt that mental deficiency presented chiefly a pedagogical, rather than mainly a medical, problem..."
- DR. MARIA MONTESSORI

CHAPTER THREE

An Overview of Autism

"I knew from the moment I saw him, something was off," says one mother about seeing her son after giving birth. Although he wasn't diagnosed with autism officially until the age of three, there were signs, she says. "He could read books forward and backwards at the age of two, but couldn't play with other children."

There are as many stories of autism as there are people living with it, each one is unique and different from the others.

Autism or Autism spectrum disorder (ASD) is a developmental disability that expresses itself in many ways, but mainly affects a person's ability to communicate and relate to others. ASD can be very severe for some, limiting communication acutely in some cases, while other individuals are high-functioning and ASD only affects them slightly. This is because Autism is a "spectrum condition," affecting individuals differently.

Over the past hundred years, the understanding of ASD has changed drastically. The name "autism" comes from the word "autos" which means self in Greek. Essentially, the word refers to someone who isolates themselves socially. While researchers and psychologists used the term to refer to symptoms of withdrawn behaviors, autism was not well defined. Until the late 1960s, it was linked to other disorders such as schizophrenia and extreme treatments such as LSD and electric shock were used.

Fortunately, there is greater understanding today, although researchers still don't know exactly what causes ASD. It does seem to run in families, and so may have to do with genetics.

Prevalence

Over the past number of years, there has been a growth in ASD diagnosis, making to be more prevalent. In reality, it's likely mostly a result of a greater awareness about ASD and improved access to diagnosis. This connection is clear when you consider the outcomes of a 2013 study. The study found that children identified with ASD were clustered in areas where greater treatment and diagnostic services were available.

The diagnosis guidelines surrounding ASD have also changed. Now, Asperger's syndrome, pervasive developmental disorders and childhood disintegrative disorder all fall under ASD. This may also explain an increase in the number of people diagnosed with ASD.

Per the CDC 2014 report, about 1 in 68 children have ASD. The disorder is more common in boys, occurring in about 1 in 54 boys. Other studies show that ASD is even more common, occurring in 1 in 45 children. These numbers may be more accurate as they're based on a parent survey rather than school records of 8-year-olds. The school records may not include students who have ASD, but aren't receiving any related special education services.

Diagnosis

Most people are diagnosed with ASD as children. While the average age of diagnosis is three, most parents report having noted symptoms earlier. The earlier the diagnosis, the earlier helpful interventions to support the child can begin.

There is no test for ASD, rather it is diagnosed using an evaluation. Usually observation is used to diagnose ASD based on criteria related to language skills, stereotypical behaviors (often repetitive or self-stimulatory behaviors) and social skills. Screening forms that parents fill out highlighting behaviors they've noticed are also useful. If you think your child may have ASD, you can ask your child's pediatrician about the process for getting an evaluation. Teachers may help notice and recommend evaluations for older children, especially in mild cases of ASD that parents may not be sure about otherwise.

ASD Symptoms

ASD mainly presents itself in difficulties interacting with others. Social skills such as interpreting body language or non-verbal communication that comes naturally to most people are difficult for people with ASD. For some, ASD means that communication is very difficult not just due to trouble with social skills, but also because they may have limited to no language skills. In other cases, people with ASD may understand speech, but be unable to produce it.

Young children may begin presenting symptoms of ASD even around the 6-month mark. Some symptoms that may be noticed in young children include:

- Little to no eye contact
- Delays in or lack of speech
- Doesn't respond to their name
- Doesn't use or react to gestures such as pointing
- Performs repetitive or self-stimulatory behaviors
- Repeats words over and over
- Severe reaction to changes in routines
- Avoids physical touch

These are only some of the symptoms, and just because you may notice some in your child doesn't necessarily mean they have ASD. Several symptoms and factors come into play when diagnosing ASD.

Another way to help track if your child may have ASD is by comparing your child's progress to developmental milestones such as saying their first word or learning to walk. While milestones serve as a guideline only and most children won't hit each milestone at the exact age listed by the CDC, it does help you get an idea of what your child should be achieving. If your child shows any significant variation from the milestones, it may indicate the presence of a developmental disorder.

Treatment

ASD is treated mainly through behavioral and language therapies. For the youngest children with ASD, early intervention programs exist to help minimize how autism affects children's abilities to interact with others and develop language skills. In addition, when entering the public-school system, an individual education plan (IEP) is created to help support the child in the classroom. Other children go to alternative schools or specially designed programs for autistic children. For children with mild forms of ASD, social skills groups and peer-mediated interventions can often be very helpful.

However, ASD treatments vary greatly from child to child because of the unique way that ASD affects each person. While there are some basic treatments (such as Applied Behavioral Analysis) that are quite popular, the same treatment doesn't produce the same results in each child. This is why parents, as advocates, play an important role in ensuring their children are getting the best treatment options for their unique needs. Trying different treatments can be helpful in finding the right balance for each child.

Children with ASD may also receive treatments for other disorders, medical conditions and symptoms as necessary. Especially for non-verbal children, it's important to look carefully for signs of other disorders, such as digestive disorders and epilepsy that are harder to detect because the child is unable to communicate.

Regardless of the treatment methods chosen and included in the child's program, the earlier parents, educators and other professionals become involved, the better the outcomes. Early intervention is one of the best ways to help your child learn new skills and reduce the need for greater interventions and assistance later.

Strengths of Individuals with ASD

ASD does not necessarily mean lower intelligence. In fact, the CDC reported that over half of children in preschool diagnosed with ASD performed above average on IQ tests.

What's more, autism has also been linked to Savant syndrome, or extraordinary abilities, even genius. There's a range of research showing that somewhere between 10 and 30% of autistic people have savant abilities. However, in the non-autistic population, the prevalence of savant abilities may be as low as 1%.

These extraordinary abilities are usually expressed in impressive mathematical abilities, an incredible memory, and artistic or musical abilities. Here are some examples:

- *Rain Man*, the movie, shows one example of an autistic person with an extraordinary memory.
- Stephen Wiltshire is an autistic artist who can fly over a city in a helicopter and then draw the cityscape from memory.
- Jacob Velasquez, who has autism, is a child piano prodigy.

Some researchers believe that there is a connection between the presence of repetitive or obsessive behaviors in ASD and extraordinary abilities. Because people on the ASD spectrum can enjoy repetitive activities for long periods of time, they may be able to practice skills longer than neurotypical people.

ASD and Other Disorders

ASD often comes along with other disorders or symptoms that aren't directly related to ASD, but are quite prevalent in people with ASD. Here are a few disorders and symptoms that commonly accompany ASD:

Sensory dysfunction

Sensory processing disorder and sensory integration disorders are some names you may hear. Sensory dysfunction affects 80-90% of people with ASD. This has commonly been associated with one of the most common behaviors seen in children and adults with ASD: self-stimulatory behavior. This behavior may involve a child wringing their hands, patting their head or clicking two objects together. One child on the autism spectrum I knew enjoyed swinging on the swings so much that he often cried when it was another child's turn. These sensory experiences are sought out by children with ASD. They may serve a purpose to calm them or relieve stress. In other cases, due to the sensory processing disorder, children may experience a need to feel their legs or other appendages. While neurotypicals know without looking that their legs are there, people with sensory disorders may feel a need to check. Placing a heavy book on the legs can help with this sensory need.

Another common trait of not looking people in the eyes may also be explained by sensory dysfunction. Some people with ASD, in addition to struggling to recognize social cues, may have a hard time looking you in the eye and listening to what you're saying at the same time. They're not trying to be rude, it's just that there's too much sensory input to pay attention to.

Digestive Troubles

Many people with ASD have very specific eating habits that may be related to a sensory disorder and their need to follow routines. For example, some people with ASD may find textures of certain foods to be very unpleasant, and so refuse to eat them. Both chronic constipation and diarrhea are more commonly found in children with ASD than in normally developing children.

ADHD

This is commonly found in people with ASD. This may be due to a genetic link.

Sleep Disorders

Up to four out of five children with autism may have chronic sleep problems. Some of these sleep problems may be related to other related disorders such as epilepsy, anxiety and digestive disorders.

Epilepsy

Between 20 and 40% of individuals with autism have epilepsy, compared to 1% of the general population.

Anxiety

People with ASD may have anxiety disorders such as social phobia and excessive worry. But, even when an actual anxiety disorder isn't present, people with ASD often show anxiety responses to certain triggers such as loud noises.

If you notice other symptoms or suspect one of these conditions in your child, it's important to get the proper diagnosis and treatment for these as well. Especially in the case of digestive troubles and epilepsy, medication can sometimes be necessary to keep things under control. Work with your child's doctor to help determine what other conditions your child may have. With a greater understanding of what your child is experiencing, you'll be able to better meet their needs.

"One test of the correctness of educational procedure is the happiness of the child."
- DR. MARIA MONTESSORI

CHAPTER FOUR

Early Intervention Using Montessori

Sprawled out on the floor, a mother plays with her 2-year-old child with ASD. The child is intently placing blocks in a straight line. The mother carefully watches and begins making her own line of blocks that runs perpendicular to her child's. They continue building until the mother's blocks run into the child's line of blocks. At a crossroads, the mother allows the child to decide how to proceed. This is a problem-solving moment.

Based on this interest in blocks, the mother may decide to introduce one of the Montessori building materials such as the pink tower, brown stairs or knobless cylinders.

These are examples of early intervention activities that may have a strong positive impact on ASD children.

In fact, the best outcomes and improvements in children with ASD are obtained through early intervention, which refers to special activities carried out with children ages 0-3. This fits in perfectly with Montessori's beliefs about education. She strongly advocated for the education of the youngest of children, even infants. According to Montessori, the younger we begin the education of children, the better.

In this chapter, we'll explore both the theoretical and practical aspects of early intervention using the Montessori method.

The Absorbent Mind

Why is early intervention better than intervening later in life? While addressing the issues and needs unique to children with ASD is important at any stage, this is especially true in their first years of life. Psychology and early childhood development hold the secrets that explain why intervention at this stage is of such great value.

Montessori, like many psychologists today, believed that childhood development is divided into stages. The first stage, from 0-3, she believed, was one of the most important. In her time, she was one of the first to truly investigate this first stage of life, which up until then had been overlooked by the medical and psychological community.

Today, we know that the first years of life are full of great brain development. It is during this stage of life that our brains are the most flexible and plastic that they will ever be. Recognizing this far before sophisticated medical equipment and tests would confirm this, Montessori described this age as "the absorbent mind." Like sponges, Montessori said, young children soaked up all the experiences and impressions gained from their environment. The richer, and greater sensory experiences provided to the child during this time, the better, she believed.

This stage of life was so important that Montessori developed a whole curriculum and philosophy for educating and caring for infants and toddlers. Within this curriculum, Montessori included activities and stimuli she believed was especially useful for infants, such as hanging mobiles above them or placing low-hanging mirrors so that they could observe themselves. She also encouraged parents to involve infants in everyday life, including chores. Even everyday activities such as going to the market or store, washing dishes and cooking were stimulating for the young mind, Montessori believed.

For children with ASD, this stage of development is of particular importance as children can learn appropriate coping mechanisms before developing their own. Experts agree that without intervention, children may begin using unhelpful or negative coping mechanisms. In addition, this is the stage where it is easiest to modify social and language practices in children with ASD.

There is evidence that people with ASD's brains are different, with connections occurring in different patterns and areas than neurotypicals. This may be another explanation for different and amazing abilities that autistic people have shown. However, for example, with social abilities and language, it's possible that a lack of development of some connections in the brain could hinder growth in these areas. Thus, what starts as a tendency or slightly different brain function grows due to the fact that interactions and behaviors that would normally develop the language and social interaction areas of the brain occur less in children with autism. During the first few years of life when the brain is very plastic, it's highly possible to alter outcomes and change these processes.

There are many kinds of intervention that are helpful for young children in "the absorbent mind" stage. Montessori's beliefs on the absorbent mind have been confirmed by scientists and researchers today. This has led to the creation of a plethora of ideas and interventions that claim to assist children with ASD. Some of the most prominent interventions with an analysis of how they may fit in with Montessori are discussed in the following two sections.

Floortime and Montessori

Floortime is an intervention used with children with ASD and other developmental disorders that was developed by Dr. Greenspan.

This intervention has been the focus of several studies and has obtained favorable outcomes for children with autism. The goal of Floortime is to create positive social connections with the parent or therapist, bring out creativity and curiosity and improve emotional development. Because social skills and emotional awareness are two areas children with autism often struggle with, it's easy to see why the method has become popular.

As the name suggests, Floortime typically takes place on the floor. Just as in the vignette that began this chapter, the adult gets on the child's level and engages in play with the child, starting with the child's interest. If the child is playing with blocks, so does the parent or therapist. If the child chooses to move a truck along the wall, the parent also chooses to play with a car. Through play, the parent or therapist gently seeks interaction with the child. Slowly, the adult pushes for more complex interactions. As children mature, Floortime can be adapted to include more difficult concepts and move into academics.

A therapist who specializes in Floortime can be a very helpful way to begin using this intervention. Therapy is often used as a time not only to interact with the child, but also to teach parents to use Floortime principles at home and continue the interventions on a day to day basis.

How does this intervention match up with Montessori principles? Quite well. Because Floortime is based on following the child's interests, which is an important component of the Montessori philosophy, it could easily be incorporated into a Montessori home or school plan. Where it may differ slightly is in the use of toys. While Montessori encourages the use of real items and avoids plastic, Floortime doesn't discourage the use of toys. However, there's no reason that natural, Montessori-style toys and materials couldn't be used in a Floortime program.

Applied Behavior Analysis and Montessori

Applied Behavior Analysis (ABA) is one of the most popular and widely used treatments for children with ASD. It's impossible to discuss ASD without addressing this treatment method. There are some cases where Montessori and ABA have been combined to help children with ASD. However, for a variety of reasons, ABA is controversial. In this section, we'll explore what ABA is and whether or not it can be used in conjunction with Montessori.

Based on B. F. Skinner's theory of operant conditioning, this method works by reinforcing certain desired behaviors. Skinner's work and development of this theory largely relied on the use of lab rats and pigeons. The animals were taught to push a lever to receive food, or taught to push a lever to stop an electrical current from shocking them. Through these "Skinner boxes" where the animals were kept, Skinner discovered that he could teach animals to follow instructions by giving them rewards and punishments.

The method of ABA itself was developed by Dr. Ole Ivar Lovaas who worked with ASD children who in many cases were unable to speak or communicate. Through rewards in the form of praise and treats (sweets, crackers, etc.) and punishments in the form of disapproval, and in some cases, even electric shocks, Lovaas reported improvements in the children's ability to speak and interact. While there has been great clinical evidence supporting the use of ABA, the experiments that have been conducted haven't met scientific standards. Despite this, there are many supporters of this method due to the results seen in the children.

Over time, the ABA method has changed drastically. Punishments are no longer commonly used in the practice, although food is still a common reward. There is a wide variety of ways to practice ABA, some that stray far from the original premise, and others that maintain closer ties to Lovaas' ideas. For example, typically, an ABA practitioner sits at a table across from the child. However, today, many practitioners sit on the floor or play on a carpet with the child, depending on their age.

From an early age, children with ASD can be treated using this method. It is popular with children of all ages on the spectrum. However, it is very intensive and there is debate whether this method is appropriate for children on the higher functioning end of ASD.

Just as there are many supporters of ABA, there are also many opponents, including a group of adults on the autism spectrum. Some of the main arguments against the use of this method include the lack of the child's ability to consent, clear discomfort shown by some children, and even the goals of ABA are drawn into question. Advocates of the rights of children with ASD argue that ABA attempts to remove autism from the child, and tries to make them the same as neurotypical children. This approach, they argue, ignores the fact that autism affects the way the brain works and that by removing autistic behaviors, ABA attempts to alter the very essence of the person.

Another common argument against ABA is that teaching the child that some behaviors are appropriate or inappropriate is based on the perceptions of non-autistic people. This is especially true in the face of self-stimulatory behaviors, which some ABA programs try to eliminate. Autism advocates argue that these behaviors are helpful and eliminate stress. Just because neurotypicals find them irritating isn't a rationale for forcing the elimination of these behaviors, they argue.

One autistic mother of a son with Asperger's, a high functioning autism spectrum disorder, notes that ABA requires children to comply with an adult at all times, resulting in extreme vulnerability. Although she didn't receive ABA treatment as a child and wasn't diagnosed until she noted differences in her son, she remarked that she was required to conform. Without blaming anyone, she shared how being forced to act in neurotypical ways "broke" her. Considering these sorts of comments made by members of the autism community, the quote included just before this chapter seems highly relevant: *"One test of the correctness of educational procedure is the happiness of the child."* Montessori believed that children could learn joyfully, without feeling "broken", extreme stress or boredom.

ABA proponents respond to these arguments claiming that ABA removes the barriers children with ASD face so that they can lead fuller lives. The ability to speak or communicate using signing or verbal language and interact with others opens their world. Some ASD adults describe feeling trapped in their younger years, unable to speak until they had success, often through ABA treatments. Other ABA practitioners such as Vince Carbone argue that we all meet certain societal norms. We all raise our children to meet certain standards, he says. "Why is it bad to do the same with autistic children?" is the question he asks.

Montessori's beliefs and the philosophy she developed can shed some further light on the controversy surrounding this treatment method. As I've already touched on by bringing up Montessori's beliefs about how learning should make children feel, the theory of ABA doesn't mesh perfectly with the Montessori philosophy. Primarily, this is because external rewards and stimulants are discouraged by the Montessori philosophy. Skinner believed that children repeat rewarded behaviors and avoid behaviors that result in negative reinforcement or punishment. Many common modern-day parenting and childcare techniques are a result of Skinner's theories. Time-out, star charts and other similar systems are all based on Skinner's work. Montessori didn't use these techniques or promote them in her philosophy. While it's difficult to say exactly what Montessori would have thought of ABA because it was developed after her death, there are many clues that can help determine whether this method can be used in combination with Montessori.

Montessori's Views on Operant Conditioning, the Basis of ABA

Overall, Montessori rejected the premise of operant conditioning and the use of rewards and punishments. Montessori did try using external rewards in her early work with children, essentially using the basics of the theory of operant conditioning. However, what she found, was that children simply wanted to work. In her words:

"..I was astonished when I learned that a child who is permitted to educate himself really gives up these lower instincts.

I then urged the teachers to cease handing out the ordinary prizes and punishments, which were no longer suited to our children, and to confine themselves to directing them gently in their work."

As you can see, Montessori ended up rejecting this model of operant conditioning. Some may even be surprised to learn that she tried this method. However, as you'll see in her beliefs about discipline, using rewards or positive reinforcement only appears to be functioning. This system doesn't cultivate the spirit of the child or help them in their search for fulfillment.

This doesn't mean that there was no discipline or method for guiding children's behavior in the classroom. Rather, it was based on different principles. To give a background to how she worked with children, it's important to understand Montessori's theory around the three levels of obedience. In her book, *The Absorbent Mind*, she devotes an entire chapter to this concept.

The first level of obedience is when the child is very young, and can only obey when what he or she wants to do coincides with what is asked of them. At times the child may obey, but it is almost as if by accident. In this stage, Montessori says, the very young child (under the age of 3) can't even obey his or her own will, let alone another's.

The second level of obedience is when a child can do what the adult asks because they recognize that it will make them happy. Herein lies the use of cajoling, rewards and punishments. While effective, this type of obedience is not the end goal. Many children end up remaining at this stage because this is all parents and teachers require of them. After all, a child doing what they're asked to do is often what teachers and parents desire. If they are happy with this result, the child is not pushed and developed further.

Montessori makes an important point in her discussion of the levels of obedience. She says, *"we must aim at cultivating the will, not at breaking it."* Through operant conditioning, the will of the individual, is essentially broken, through teaching the individual to change their will or to want and desire something else. Think of it this way, children are often rewarded for sitting still and being quiet at school, but, children don't actually want to sit still and be quiet. They'd rather be in movement, become completely engrossed in a project or activity and speak to their friends as necessary. By rewarding children for sitting quietly, we change their will. However, in Montessori's method, children can move and are able to find meaningful activities and projects to concentrate on. Perhaps the results are similar, a quiet, orderly classroom, but in one, the child's will has been broken and in the other, the child's will has been cultivated to seek and carry out work.

This brings us to the third level of obedience. In this level, the child obeys because they see the value in what's been requested of them, and so joyfully comply. In other words, as Montessori quotes a child answering the question *"So this is the school where you do as you like?"* the child says *"No, ma'am...it is not that we do as we like, but we like what we do."* This child understood the value of deciding to do something, and then doing it. At this stage, the child chooses to participate fully in the community, find meaningful work and happily meet the norms within the classroom because they are good. Of course, this is partially dependent on having an excellent guide or teacher who knows what to ask of the children. Should the teacher greatly limit the freedoms of the children, this level of obedience is nearly impossible to achieve.

So, what did Montessori do to encourage the development all the way to the third level of obedience? Montessori used many tools to develop the character and "spirit", as she called it, of the children she worked with. Encouraging independence, using routines, allowing children to be in charge of cleaning the classrooms, freedom of choice and following the child are some of the main principles Montessori used in her classrooms.

Another important tool popular in Montessori classrooms is the use of descriptive praise. This is a form of praise that, contrary to evaluative praise, helps children internalize the positive aspects of their behavior or decisions. Typical evaluative praise, which can be used as positive feedback in operant conditioning, sounds like this: "good girl!" "good boy!" "good job!" "great job!" "excellent!" You may be wondering, what's wrong with that?

The problem is that adults are typically the ones who decide whether the child's behavior, work or even their whole being is "good" rather than "bad." This can leave the child feeling helpless, as this arbitrary evaluation doesn't lie in their hands. How can you get more praise like this? By being "good", but what is "good"? It's not explicit.

With descriptive praise like "I saw you worked hard," or "Way to keep a positive attitude," on the other hand, praises things children have more control over. Children can then internalize these behaviors and recognize their value. Descriptive praise also helps children see the benefit of their efforts. For example, if you thank a child for cleaning, you can say "Thanks for wiping up that mess. Now the table is clean for someone else to use." This further helps the child reach the third stage of obedience, because the value of the work they've done is highlighted.

In addition, Montessori used discipline measures that still respected the child and their needs, but enforced limits. A child acting out in the classroom might be invited to sit closer to the teacher, for example, rather than sending them away. This proximity to the teacher allows the child to observe other children working, see a new lesson, and also feel the security that the teacher offers. These sorts of measures, rather than seen as punishments, are simply meeting the child's needs for support, quiet or an opportunity to refocus themselves.

Although the former discipline techniques may work well with children with ASD, what about descriptive praise? Wouldn't this be an overwhelming or worthless technique for children with limited language skills? Let's explore some additional possibilities and Montessori's work with children on the ASD spectrum.

A Case for a Mix of ABA and Montessori

When referring to children with ASD, the purpose of ABA changes, and the goals of operant conditioning are more related to encouraging socialization or the use of language rather than discipline related issues. It is difficult to say whether Montessori would have used ABA with children on the spectrum.

In her earliest work, Montessori probably did work with children on the ASD spectrum. It was in this work that she began developing her method and creating her first original learning materials. In her works, you can see how she highlights the scientific process. She encourages teachers to observe their students in detail and try new methods with them to see what's successful and what's not. Through this method, she achieved impressive results. Children who had been shut away in institutions with mentally ill adults were able to read, communicate and participate actively in life with her help.

Some Montessorians have taken this focus on the scientific method as an invitation to try new techniques in tandem with traditional Montessori activities. One such person is Michelle Lane. An ABA expert turned Montessorian, Michelle Lane began and ran her own Montessori school called the Lane Montessori School for Autism, which was a non-profit organization that unfortunately closed in 2010 due to lack of funds. However, she continues to research and share her extensive knowledge and experiences from beginning and running the first combined ABA and Montessori school in the world.

Using all of the traditional Montessori materials, classroom preparation guidelines and philosophy, Lane also made use of ABA. In an interview with blogger Lori Bourne from *Montessori for Everyone*, Lane shared some insights into how she combined the two methods. When discussing the school, Lane said "*It is similar only in terms of the curriculum and classroom layout...The difference is how we teach. We work one-to-one, with prompting and reinforcement schedules based on each step of the task analysis. In addition, we have set programs/activities that the child must do each day.*" The "reinforcement schedule" refers to the ABA component. This language suggests that children may have been given treats or verbal positive reinforcement at different stages throughout a Montessori activity. Children at Lane's school "*responded even better than I had imagined,*" suggesting that the combination has the potential to help many children with ASD.

In the end, it's up for each parent to decide what's best for their child. While some may decide after trying ABA that it's an integral part of their child's life, others may decide not to try it at all. As mentioned before, each child is different and what is a perfect solution for one child may not be appropriate for another. It's up to parents to make the decision and respond to their child in the way they feel is best.

Montessori Early Intervention Activities for ASD

The Montessori method, as mentioned previously, had its beginnings with students with special needs. Because the same diagnostic tests and names for disorders didn't exist at the time that Montessori worked with these children, we can't be sure if she worked with ASD children, although it's highly likely. In any case, her approach can be very effective with ASD children.

Many of the traditional Montessori activities can be used with ASD students. Before we get into listing some of the most appropriate activities to use, I want to make a quick note about following the child. We'll get into this in detail in some of the upcoming chapters, but as you're reading through these activities, remember to observe your child. Notice what they seem to enjoy most and try to follow their interests. In Montessori, repetition is welcome. Allow your child to repeat activities as desired.

In addition, try using descriptive praise with your child, or use a positive response such as a smile or hug to share your child's success and encourage them to continue employing their efforts when engaging in these activities. If you decide to include Floortime or ABA therapies, you may want to speak with an experienced therapist who can provide guidance for how to incorporate these interventions into your Montessori plans.

Here are some ideal Montessori activities for early intervention for children with ASD.

Sensory Basket

Fill a basket with a few items surrounding a theme. Ideally, these items should be natural. For example, a few different types of balls made with different fabrics, or perhaps a few made of wood or wicker. Or you could make up a basket with laminated photos of farm animals. Another theme could be color. Make up a white basket with a white seashell, a feather, a piece of wool or cotton, some white lace, and a white stone, etc. The idea behind these baskets is for little ones to explore using their senses. Baskets should include a variety of different textures, colors, images and noises. Make sure that all objects are safe and that you supervise your child when using the baskets, as children at this age are likely to place objects in their mouth.

You can set up a low shelf in your child's room or another area of your home and place one or two baskets for your child to explore as desired. You might even consider using the objects to sing a song with your child, such as "Old MacDonald" with the farm animal pictures.

Stringing Beads

Place some large beads in a basket with a shoe-string. Demonstrate how to string the beads onto the shoe-string. Then, invite your child to try. Many children enjoy repeating this activity over and over again. It's a great way to develop fine motor skills.

Pink Tower

The pink tower is a very famous Montessori material ideal for the youngest students. Composed of 10 cubes ranging from 1 cm^3 to 10 cm^3, the pink tower teaches the concept of base ten. The goal is for children to learn to build the tower by stacking the cubes on top of each other, largest to smallest. Weight and size help guide children as they work on this.

As a parent or teacher, it's important to demonstrate how to use the tower. Using two hands, and without using any words, carefully move each cube to the work area. Then, using two hands to feel weight and sizes, determine which is the largest. Slowly and deliberately work on building the tower, allowing the child to get involved if they are interested.

Practical Life Activities

These activities should be the backbone of early intervention. Montessori especially advocated for these activities among the youngest of children. They help children develop self-esteem, independence and a sense of belonging. Practical life activities are simply a more intentional way of involving your child in everyday chores and tasks around the home. Here are some examples:

- **Food Preparation**

    For the youngest, something as simple as cutting a banana with a butter knife can be rewarding and fun. You can make these activities extra exciting for your child by including their favorite foods. Large slices of watermelon lend themselves to the use of cookie cutters. Or, allow your young child to spread cream cheese or peanut butter on a piece of toast. As with all Montessori presentations, first demonstrate, and then allow your child to try. Then enjoy eating the snack together!

    As your child develops interest and skills in this area, you can also use a small, child-sized table and ask your child to help you place a table cloth on it. Set out plates and take your snack to the table to enjoy together. A small pitcher can be provided for your little one to practice serving water.

- **Hygiene**

    Create a space in your bathroom or your child's room where they can practice personal hygiene activities. Use a step stool in the bathroom and teach your child to wash their hands. Put a mirror at your child's level. Provide a comb or brush and show your child how to brush their hair. Other activities include washing their face, brushing teeth and even getting dressed independently.

- **Cleaning**

    Invite your child to participate in cleaning activities. This can include washing dishes, wiping down tables, sweeping and more. Try to be creative in making it possible for your child to participate independently. For example, purchase a child-sized broom. For washing dishes, place two basins, one for washing and one for rinsing on a child sized table, or use a safe step-stool so that your child can reach the sink. Remember to place a large towel to catch any spilled water, assuring that this doesn't interfere with the step-stool.

- **Gardening**

    A wonderful sensorial experience, gardening provides an opportunity for children to get closer to nature and feel the calm this offers. Invite your child to plant seeds and seedlings, weed and water in the garden. Consider planting herbs and inviting your child to smell the different scents. Encourage your child to get into it. Just plan a bath afterwards.

    Some children may feel an aversion to getting dirty. If this is the case, try allowing your child to observe, or provide gloves, tools and a blanket to sit on so they can avoid getting too dirty. Or, invite your child to participate in watering indoor plants as they grow comfortable with the idea.

3 Period Lesson

This fundamental Montessori lesson is wonderful for helping your child develop language skills. You can use this lesson with picture cards or objects. For example, consider things you have around the home such as fruit. Present your child with 3 different whole fruits on a table or carpet. Choose fruit that looks very different from each other, such as an apple, an orange, a banana, grapes or a lemon.

In the first period of the lesson, you'll name each of the fruits, pointing to each one. Encourage your child to try to say the names. Then, in the second period, you'll ask your child to point to or pick up the fruit you name. Finally, in the third period, you point to the fruit and ask your child to say the name.

For the youngest children, you can omit the third period all together. It's important for children to show mastery in period 2 before moving on to period 3. And remember, you want your child to feel successful. If your child starts acting very frustrated, consider going back to period one, and offering your child a taste of each fruit while naming them. You can end the lesson there and try again another day.

Gross Motor Activities

From the time babies are born, they feel a need to move. First in jerking movements, then in coordinated crawling, babies are driven to develop their gross motor skills. This continues throughout childhood. Montessori encouraged parents and teachers to include gross motor activities in the classroom and allow children to have plenty of time to exercise. Some Montessori activities you can try include:

- **Walking the Circle**

    Using masking or painter's tape, tape a large circle on a floor. Show your child how to walk around the circle, stepping on the tape. Then, you can invite your child to increase the difficulty by carrying a basket or cup of beans while walking. Or, use a bean bag for them to balance on their head.

- **Moving Furniture**

    Montessori was one of the first educators to suggest using child-sized furniture. In doing so, her goal was not only to make children feel comfortable. She also recognized that children would be able to move the furniture in the classroom. This provides great gross motor practice and real natural consequences. Providing your child with light, wooden child-sized furniture will provide your child with opportunities for moving chairs, tables and stools. This provides great gross motor practice.

If any of these activities seems too big and overwhelming, try breaking it down into parts. For example, present only three of the Pink Tower blocks at a time. Or, only go through a few steps of a lesson at a time. Slowly, but surely, you can help your child build on their abilities.

"Scientific observation then has established that education is not what the teacher gives; education is a natural process spontaneously carried out by the human individual, and is acquired not by listening to words but by experiences upon the environment."
- DR. MARIA MONTESSORI

Chapter Five

Montessori Sensorial Experiences and Autism

On playground duty one day, a boy with autism from my class ran up behind me and gave me a big hug. He nuzzled up against me and jumped up and down, rubbing his head on my arm. I scratched his back and he made joyful noises in delight. Contact was important for him at that stage. Although he could be protective of his space at times, he often sought out a hug or a back scratch. He also chewed on his finger, a self-stimulatory behavior, to the point that he had a large callous on it. As I recall, sensory experiences could be very calming for him.

Another boy at the school was known for his uncanny listening ability. Also on the autism spectrum, this boy could match the Montessori sound cylinders more accurately than most of the teachers, being a particularly challenging set of cylinders. He was thrilled at his ability to excel in this area.

In both of these examples, the senses and sensory experiences were important. For these children, the senses of touch and hearing were sources of comfort. In the classroom, and in their lives, recognizing and building on this was a positive and helpful way to direct learning.

One of the unique points in Montessori education, especially for young children, is an emphasis on sensorial experiences. For autistic children, the senses are important. As mentioned in chapter 2, self-stimulatory behavior is a common occurrence in children living with ASD. Sensory dysfunction is also common in children with ASD. The use of senses in educational activities can help children with autism improve their response to sensory stimuli. Furthermore, Montessori believed that children in general learned through hands-on, sensory-rich experiences. In contrast to the sit down, lecture and dictation style of learning that was common in schools in her day, Montessori knew that children learn by doing.

What does this mean? Although the latest craze you'll see on any Pinterest board related to early childhood and sensory experiences is reminiscent of Montessori, the approach is a bit more refined in the Montessori method. To clarify, creating sensory boxes, allowing your child to squeeze and enjoy cool, cooked spaghetti, water play and other sensory activities are great. However, in the Montessori method, especially for children age 0-6, there are some very specific materials and lessons that can be used with great benefit for children.

In this chapter, benefits of the use of sensory materials and activities will be discussed. Then, some practical applications and activity suggestions for children over a range of ages are offered.

Benefits of Sensorial Activities

There are many benefits to be gained from sensory activities. Many children view these activities as "fun" because they allow for movement, something that children crave, and often take a unique approach to the senses that is often left out in everyday life.

Here are some of the main benefits:

Hands-On

Sensorial activities focus on the use of materials that are to be moved around and used in a hands-on way. This can be challenging for some ASD children with tactile system dysfunction, which makes touching objects, especially of different textures, uncomfortable. Others, however, get great pleasure from touching these sorts of objects. In either case, these activities can be helpful in teaching the brain to respond to different tactile sensory input. As Sally J Rogers and Geraldine Dawson outline in their book *Early Start Denver Model for Young Children with Autism*, by changing the input given to the brain, different pathways and weak areas can be stimulated. Through these changes, it may be possible to develop a stronger ability to receive sensory input and organize it in the brain.

Hands-on activities and experiences are also known to create stronger memories. The more senses included in the learning experience, the better. Have you ever been taken back in time, just through a smell? Perhaps you smell baking bread and remember how your mother baked bread when you were a child. For learning, using the senses is a way to create stronger memories and connections in the brain.

Language Skills

The focus is on the materials, and speaking is minimal. This allows students with ASD to isolate vocabulary and reduces the possibility that they may be overwhelmed by auditory input. Furthermore, language skills may be developed as students are able to focus on acquiring specific words related to the presentation. For example, a presentation on textures provides the opportunity to learn words such as "rough" and "smooth".

Boost in Self-Confidence

As I mentioned, many autistic children may have a sensitivity to a certain sense, allowing them to perform very well using the materials. This can help instill self-confidence and a positive self-image in the child. Creating a positive and encouraging learning environment where the child feels successful is vital to helping engage them in other, more challenging areas.

Montessori Sensorial Activities

Traditionally, the Montessori sensorial activities are introduced with children ages 0-6. In the primary classroom (ages 3-6), many of these activities lay the base for the fundamentals of understanding math and numbers. However, many others of the activities are aimed at what Montessori called "the education of the senses." In *The Absorbent Mind*, Montessori writes:

"Our sensorial material provides a kind of guide to observation, for it classifies the impressions that each sense can receive: the colors, notes, noises, forms and sizes, touch-sensations, odors and tastes. This undoubtedly is also a form of culture, for it leads us to pay attention both to ourselves and to our surroundings."

By guiding children to observe intently, we are setting them up for an increased ability to concentrate, notice important details and fully participate in life. For children on the ASD spectrum, the use of sensorial materials may even affirm some of their strongest tendencies and inclinations towards the senses. And for others, it helps them develop a way to organize sensory information by isolating each sense.

As you approach these sensory activities, remember to be aware of your child's needs. As discussed, many children have sensory sensitivities that make certain sensory activities either highly desirable or uncomfortable. If your child reacts in a very negative way, you can simply end the activity and try a different one. Here they are:

Auditory

Sound Cylinders

These wooden cylinders typically include 6 different sounds in two equal sets for a total of 12 cylinders. Similar to rattles, the cylinders are filled with different materials (that are invisible to the child) that range from a very soft sound to a loud sound. Two different colors are typically used to denote each set of cylinders, for example red and blue. The goal is for children to find each cylinder's match. In a demonstration, the teacher or parent shows the child how to line up the cylinders in two vertical columns. Then, selecting a cylinder from the left-hand set, shake it near your ear. Then, taking a cylinder from the right-hand set, shake it near your right ear. Compare to the cylinder from the right-hand set to the one you had picked up from the left-hand set. Continue comparing with the different cylinders from the right-hand set until you find a match. Then, invite the child to try matching. Continue working methodically until all matches are found.

Bells

Just as with the wooden cylinders, a set of bells is used for students to use to match tones. This material is attractive for many children as they can also learn to play songs using the bells.

Olfactory

Smelling Bottles

The smelling bottles are similar to the sound cylinders. Except, as you can imagine, instead of sounds in the cylinders, there are smells. Typically, very strong, easily identifiable scents are used such as mint, cinnamon, oregano, ginger, vanilla, etc. You can make your own bottles using essential oils as long as there are no visual cues that would help your child with the task. The goal of the task is to match the scents that are the same.

Taste

Tasting Bottles

Tasting bottles are also similar to the smelling bottles and sound cylinders. Using a dropper, different tastes can be tried. In this task, the child is encouraged to match tastes that are the same. However, you can also do a similar activity by blindfolding your child and offering different fruits, and asking your child to guess the name of the fruit.

Tactile Sense

There are many activities that focus on the tactile sense. Here are a few examples with short descriptions:

Rough and Smooth Boards and Grading Tablets

These materials were developed to teach about textures, but also the language and vocabulary that's used to describe them. First, the rough and smooth boards are used to teach the difference between rough and smooth. These boards consist of a smooth wooden board with strips of sand paper placed at equal spaces along the board. The child strokes the smooth board, then the rough sandpaper, and so on until reaching the end of the board. In a demonstration, the guide states the vocabulary while touching the board. The child is then invited to try.

The second material, the grading tablets, have different grades of sandpaper, ranging from very fine-bit to very rough. In a first demonstration, only one set of the tablets is used. First, a demonstration shows the blindfolded guide stroking all the tablets and organizing them from smooth to rough. Vocabulary such as "rough", "rougher", and "the roughest" is used. As a follow-up presentation, the child can be presented with two sets of the tablets and asked to match the textures that are the same. A visual check afterwards can help children determine whether they matched correctly.

Fabric Box

You can easily make this material on your own. The premise here is to introduce new textures in two sets of about 5 different materials, just as with the graded tablets. Cut out squares of uniquely textured fabric. Some good options are: jeans, velvet, silk, polyester, wool, felt. Make sure you get 2 squares of each material so that you can practice matching the sets with your child. Use a blindfold to do this work. You can check if you got them right by looking at your matches afterwards.

Pressure Cylinders

This material is similar to the others mentioned in that it requires matching of two different sets. The material features two sets of cylinders (identifiable by color). On top of each cylinder is a button that can be pressed down with the thumb. However, each one requires a different amount of pressure to get it down. This material can require some practice to get used to. Consider adding colored dots on the bottom as a control of error so children know if they've matched the cylinders correctly.

Sensory Walking Tiles

Purely for a fun experience, sensory walking tiles can be created for children to walk over with bare feet. Consider making them yourself using deep trays. Some materials you might use include cotton balls, sand, wood chips, rice, smooth river stones and others. In addition to stimulating the tactile system, the walking tiles also engage the vestibular system, or our balance system present in the inner ear. Many ASD children experience dysfunctions with the vestibular system. Balancing exercises such as walking over different materials such as sensory tiles can help strengthen this system.

Thermic Sense

Thermic Tablets

These matching and grading tablets are made from a range of different materials that feel cold or warm to the touch. For example, slate feels cooler than cork or felt and steel is colder still. Encouraging children to feel and grade these different thermal sensations helps develop concentration and heightens sensory awareness.

Stereognostic Sense

Geometric Solids

The 3D shapes we all know such as a cube, and sphere come to life in the geometric solids. Children are invited to learn these shapes by touch and by name. First children are invited to touch each of the solids. Children notice which solids slide, roll or slide and roll (such as a cone). Different activities including classification, naming and matching to solid plane figures are completed using these figures. Many children also enjoy building with these figures and experimenting with what they can do. Some traditional Montessorians prefer to use the materials strictly for the purposes of the planned presentations, however others allow for more experimental play. It's up to you to decide what approach to take.

The Mystery Bag

This fun activity allows children to use their stereognostic sense. This is what allows us to identify an object just by touching it, without seeing it. In a typical mystery bag, two sets of identical objects are provided. Half are in the bag and half are outside. Without looking, the child holds one object from outside the bag in one hand and searches for the matching object in the bag with the other hand. It's best to start out with only a few objects (3 or 4) and then build up to larger sets. Although this material is available for purchase using geometrical solids made of wood, you could also make your own set using household objects.

Visual

Color Tablets

The color tablets can be used for a wide range of activities. There are 3 Color Boxes for purchase. However, they can easily be made on your own using buttons for boxes 1 and 2, and paint sample cards for box 3. Typically, children begin by matching primary colors to primary colors using box 1. In a basket, two of each primary color are presented, and then mixed up. After a demonstration, the child is invited to match the colors. Then, more colors are added to practice matching using box 2

Then, grading of color hues can be presented to children using the color box 3. In my experience, it's best to start with just 4 of the graded tablets from the black to white set. Demonstrate arranging them from light to dark. Then, other sets of colors can be introduced. Finally, the full gradation of 7 tablets can be presented.

Knobbed cylinders

Showing differences in diameter, depth and weight, these cylinders challenge students to find the right match. Like a puzzle, cylinders with small knobs are removed from the base, and then replaced. There are four different blocks, each emphasizing the different aspects in a unique way. One of the reasons Montessori created this material was to help young children learn to grip a pencil properly. By strengthening the pincer grip through use of the knobbed cylinders, children can improve their fine motor skills in preparation for writing activities. Many ASD children struggle with fine motor control, related to a dysfunction in the proprioceptive system, which is part of the sensory system. This, and many of the other sensorial materials and practical life activities can help children strengthen this system, improving fine motor control.

Knobless cylinders

Using the same dimensions and concepts of varying diameter, height and weight, these cylinders also come in 4 colored sets. However, they are not knobbed and do not come with a base. These cylinders are used for building towers and creating different designs. These cylinder sets are often used in combination for different exercises. Due to their small size, very precise movements are needed for children to be able to stand them up.

Pink Tower

This material was described in the previous chapter, but it is still a valuable material to use with older children. If your child has mastered the use of this material, consider adding the brown stair (below) and using the two in combined creations.

Brown Stair

The brown stair uses the same concept as the pink tower, but the pieces are rectangular prisms rather than cubes. The same dimensions are used, so the pink tower can be laid out along-side the brown stair and they match perfectly. Again, this material helps prepare children for understanding quantities and numbers, while also encouraging gross and fine motor development.

Red Rods

The red rods are another material that are a precursor to understanding numbers. Ten rods in incremental sizes are provided. In addition to placing them in order, children can use the rods to practice measuring, learn vocabulary such as "long", "short", "longer", "longest", "shorter", and "shortest." Another activity involves creating a maze to walk through using the material.

As you can see, the sensorial materials are varied and enticing for children to use. The great variety doesn't suggest that you need to use all of them, however exposing your child to a wide variety can help you identify interests, strengths and weaknesses. As you explore with your child, notice their favorite materials. Most of these materials include a basic presentation which can be followed up on with extensions, or more challenging activities. For example, an extension for the fabric box might involve learning the names of the different types of cloth.

An older student may even learn how each type of material is made, which could in turn become a geography project or a lesson in biology, studying silkworms. The possibilities are endless for taking sensorial materials to the next level. This way, you can continue to create stimulating activities based on sensory experiences for your child even as they grow and mature.

"Education should no longer be mostly imparting of knowledge, but must take a new path, seeking the release of human potential."
- DR. MARIA MONTESSORI

CHAPTER SIX

Following the Child and Autism

"No, no, no," he cried. "I don't like English."

"I know," I replied calmly. "Let's work with these cards." I said, showing him the cards. David, an ASD student, whose native language was Spanish, resisted working with me in English. But, I had noticed he liked working with some cards the Spanish-speaking teacher had made to match words and pictures. His therapist had also suggested he might enjoy working with pictures rather than words alone. This fit in well to the Montessori method, but he was beyond the one-word Pink Material cards used for beginning reading. But even the earliest reader books we had seemed challenging. So, I had made up some cards using rhyming consonant-vowel-consonant words like "cat, sat, fat, etc." into silly sentences like "The fat cat sat on a bat." I drew pictures to go along with them. They were kind of amusing and fun.

After seeing the cards, David seemed more willing to work with me. We looked at the pictures and read the cards together, matching each written card to the correct picture card. Over the next few weeks, he returned to the cards again and again. Other children in the class also enjoyed them.

With David, I had learned that for him to feel calm and ready to work I needed to follow his lead carefully. His ASD manifested itself in a certain level of anxiety, especially when it came to getting out of his comfort zone and practicing new skills such as English. By following his interests, strengths and trying to understand his mood, we were often able to work well together.

One of the pillars of the Montessori method is to follow the child. There are many reasons that she developed this guideline for her method. For children on the ASD spectrum and neurotypical children alike, there is much to be gained by following this key component of the method.

In this chapter, we'll cover some of the important areas that following the child touches upon, especially with regards to education and children with ASD. Then, some guidelines will be offered to help you as you seek to find a balance between following your child and guiding them on their journey to greater independence and personal and academic achievements.

Why is Following the Child Important

There are many benefits to be gained from following the child in their interests. What does this mean exactly? In part, it means that rather than the adult choosing activities based on what they'd like to see the child learn, they observe the child to discover what it is they are interested in learning.

Think about it. Let's imagine you choose a new activity or skill to learn. You decide that you'd like to take an oil painting class. You've always wanted to learn, but have never had the chance. So, you go to the community center to sign up and they say that they think you should take a basic mechanics class. You don't want to learn about mechanics, but they send you up to the class anyway. The whole time you're there, you can't help but daydream about being in an art class instead. So, you don't learn very much in the mechanics class and end up sort of frustrated. You quit the class and go find an art studio across town where you begin your oil painting class. Because you're so excited about it, you apply yourself and soak up every minute. By the end of the course, you've mastered the basic concepts of oil painting and have completed several paintings.

Just like we have our own unique interests and motivations, so do our children. Who knows, maybe someday you'll consider the practical aspects of the mechanics class and decide to take it, but it wasn't what you wanted at the time. Can you imagine how frustrated your child feels when they are drawn to master a certain skill or learn about a topic, and they are forced to learn something else?

By following our child's interests, we can take advantage of all the motivation and energy that they're ready to use towards mastering a new skill. This is one of the principal benefits of following the child: achievement and mastery of skills, both academic and non-academic.

Following the child truly allows them to fully express their sensitive periods as well. What are sensitive periods?

Sensitive Periods

Sensitive periods are similar to milestones. However, it's a concept that can help you understand your child well beyond toddlerhood when most parents stop following milestones.

Sensitive periods refer to a period when a child concentrates on achieving a certain skill. Typically, babies have a sensitive period for movement and walking from the time they're born until they are stable walkers. Any parent knows that a child will demand to be allowed to practice walking during a certain period of time. They struggle, fall, get up and fight until they master this skill. This sensitive period for movement is one that all parents must understand because most children are so insistent on communicating this need that they must walk. So, back bent over, parents hold their child's hand, encourage and help their small child.

Similar sensitive periods occur throughout childhood. While many, like milestones, can be predicted to happen around a certain time, or a certain age, others are not so predictable. For example, Montessori believed that the sensitive period for language is between birth and the age of 6. This is a pretty wide age-range. It is during this time that children show great interest in learning new words, learning to speak and even may show interest in beginning to read and write.

If you look at your child's interests through this lens, you may find yourself more understanding of their sometimes quirky behavior. Children often demand their independence, striving to do things "all by myself" because of a great need to master a skill.

While children on the ASD spectrum may differ from neurotypical children in when they begin reaching milestones or experiencing sensitive periods, they also express many of the same interests and need to master skills.

With regards to sensitive periods, Montessori viewed them as windows of opportunity. For example, due to the sensitive period for language from birth to age 6, caregivers should take advantage to expose the child to an extensive vocabulary now. This is why she included nomenclature (or 3-part) cards in her preschool curriculum. These cards teach everything from the vocabulary of the anatomy of animals to botanical vocabulary, the names of household items and more.

By carefully observing your child and studying their sensitive periods, you can be prepared to support their learning. Just like in the example of the painting class, rather than forcing a class in mechanics, you can offer a wonderful oil painting class and studio with all the necessary supplies to work with. Your child is sure to respond in a positive way and through their motivation and interest, achieve mastery much more quickly than if you diverted their interests down other paths.

Pace

Following the child removes some of the pressure of "keeping up" with the class, or in a home setting, "keeping up" with what other kids your child's age are doing. By following the child, you simply move at their pace and introduce new skills and ideas as your child masters others. The level of challenge increases over time and activities are perfectly adequate for the child's level.

In the Montessori classroom, the norm is that each child moves at their pace through the curriculum. While some might learn to read at an age that's traditionally considered early, others might do so later than convention typically accepts. But, in both cases, the pace of the child is respected. Because children are allowed to select their own interests (although guidance is provided), children aren't forced to follow any certain plan that will ensure they're reading, writing or adding by a certain age.

Lois Omonde, a one-on-one aid to an ASD student in a Montessori upper-elementary classroom, commented *"He...learned at his own pace. Writing was hard for him. We modified a lot of lessons including using the computer to write. He was able to access much of the same curriculum as the other students his age."* This is only one example, but as you can see in this case, even without pushing the student, he was able to make use of the same curriculum as his peers. The point isn't whether students are doing things that others their age can do. Rather, the point is that all children have an incredible built-in desire and motivation to learn. With the right tools, modifications and by following them, they can achieve great things. We don't have to push them to do so.

It's impossible to talk about pace without considering the rest of society. It can be hard to communicate that you're following your child's pace to others who would have you push them to meet certain standards or hold them back. Stay firm in your decision. In following your child and carefully guiding their learning across academics, practical life skills and grace and courtesy skills, your child is sure to progress.

Behavior

Another reason that following the child is important relates to behavior. Montessori believed that no behavior expressed by the child was without meaning. Rather, she thought that children communicated through their behavior. An angry, frustrated or bored child may communicate by acting out or doing something naughty.

Montessori said that *"The children in our schools have proved to us that their real wish is to always be at work."* She notes that in her experience, children act out mainly out of *"insufficient nourishment of the life of the mind."* However, providing interesting activities isn't enough. Montessori believed that there are impediments that can diminish a child's ability to fully participate in their mental life.

One of these impediments is the child's ability to concentrate. Through practical life activities, Montessori encouraged children to develop a sense of order and increase their ability to concentrate.

A second impediment is us. As adults, we often, either out of good intentions or impatience, interfere with what our children are doing. Another famous Montessori quote, which is one to live by, is *"never help a child with a task at which he feels he can succeed."* Unless the child asks for help or becomes too frustrated and cries, there's absolutely no reason to get involved. While we might notice the struggle, and wish to help, the struggle is where all the action is. It's where the learning is happening. To truly follow your child, you must allow them to complete tasks, even if you cringe from afar.

For example, you might have a hard time watching your child wrestle with a container to open it. Perhaps pretzels will even go flying everywhere after your child abruptly opens it. However, this creates an opportunity for your child to learn. After watching this, a wise Montessori parent would offer an activity featuring different types of containers with lids and some objects to place inside as a lesson.

Back to the point, our children often express themselves in confusing ways and undesired behaviors. However, Montessori shows us that many behavior problems may be a result of a need to do work that the child enjoys. I have often noticed this pattern in my own children. They may be in the beginning stages of a tantrum. Often it can be avoided by directing their attention to an interesting project or activity that I know they're excited about. My nearly 2-year-old loves stringing beads. Whenever she's bothering her older brother who may be engrossed in an art project, she can often be happily diverted to this activity. Her interest in her brother's project is often an indication that she wants something special to do, too.

Of course, there are other reasons for bad behavior. Hunger, fatigue, frustration, sensory triggers, sadness and a need for connection with a parent or caregiver are also sometimes expressed in undesired behaviors. As parents and caregivers, it's our role to seek to understand all behavior and try to fulfill those deeper needs that may not always be visible on the surface.

Guidelines for Following Your Child with ASD

Following your child with ASD is a challenging, but rewarding journey. Here are some practical guidelines for following your child:

Observe First

Before you immediately react to what your child is doing (unless it's obviously dangerous, like touching a fire), observe. Notice what your child is doing, what objects they're using and try to imagine their goal, or the reason that they may be doing something.

Self-stimulatory behaviors are a perfect example of this. Although my first impulse with David, my student with ASD who often gnawed on his finger was to ask him to stop, or look me in the eyes, I realized that he needed to chew on something and that looking me in the eye was uncomfortable or distracting for him.

There are many examples of children, with ASD or not, who need to fidget and move. A large rubber band placed on a chair for the child to push with their legs against, or a stress ball to pinch and press are some easy solutions that may provide the relief in movement your child needs.

Whenever you see your child engaging in a behavior, whether positive or negative, try to remain impartial and understand the behavior before reacting.

Follow Montessori's Rule

This brings us to Montessori's rule about not interfering with tasks your child feels they can succeed at. Once you've observed, try to refrain from interfering as long as your child feels they will succeed. I admit, I used to feel an urge to intervene when I noticed my oldest child making a mess out of watering the flowers, getting himself completely soaked and muddy. Now, I just make sure he knows how to clean up. Over the years, he's gotten better at it and no longer gets soaked head to toe.

Most parents will run into similar situations in which their child attempts to do something, and makes a complete mess of it. Rather than stopping this impulse of action, I've learned to let children continue in their work.

In the same way, even if your child is succeeding in a difficult task, you should also avoid intervening. Montessori says *"Praise, help, or even a look, may be enough to interrupt him, or destroy the activity. It seems a strange thing to say, but this can happen even if the child merely becomes aware of being watched."* It's understandable. Most adults also seek solitude to concentrate and feel interrupted when someone walks into the room as we're in the middle of a difficult task. Wait until your child has finished the activity to comment on what has been accomplished.

So, how can you plan for this in your life? This means giving our child plenty of warning before you go somewhere. This will help ensure that there's enough time for them to do simple tasks like getting their shoes and jacket on by themselves. For older children, it might mean making time and space for them to help make their school lunch or do their own laundry. By encouraging this independence and allowing children to complete tasks on their own, children gain self-confidence and advance in their abilities.

To truly fulfill this rule of Montessori's, most parents and teachers also need to retrain themselves. Just a quick look out of the corner of your eye can let you know your child is attempting to put their shoes on by themselves After noticing this, you can go on with whatever you're doing until they either complete the task successfully or ask for help (either by asking or crying). You'll get better at this as you practice and make a habit out of not interrupting your concentrating child as much.

Build Concentration

Many children, with or without ASD, struggle to concentrate. One child with ASD at the school where I worked would use one material during nearly the whole work time, but not because he was concentrating on using the material correctly. Rather, he would use the pieces and invent his own little world, imagining blocks were airplanes or little people moving around. This prevented him from participating in any work that challenged him and allowed him to develop new skills.

Other children with ASD may stare into space, seemingly shutting themselves off from everything else in the room. One girl with ASD I knew would often seem to be daydreaming. After calling her name, she would be completely startled, and ask "What? What happened?"

However, through engaging activities, we can help build concentration that is useful for all kinds of learning. One favorite activity for the girl I mentioned was cleaning the fish tank. She fully participated in this and enjoyed thoroughly brushing the moss and sliminess off the stones before filling the tank with fresh water and returning the fish.

Practical life activities like cleaning the fish tank are often ideal for helping children develop concentration. However, the key is really to follow your child, find their interest, and choose the activity based on this.

Find an Appropriate Outlet

Sometimes you may find your child expressing a need in an inappropriate way. For example, running back and forth inside the house, yelling, hiding under the table, playing with water for a long time at the sink when it's time to wash hands are all examples of a child expressing a need. In the water example, the child may be expressing a need to play with water. By allowing a longer bath-time or creating a space to experiment with water in the kitchen, you can give your child an outlet for their needs. Hiding under the table may show a need for a dark, solitary place to spend time, such as small tent or cave of sorts that could easily be made for your child in their room.

Although frustrating at times, viewing a child's behavior in this light can help us show empathy towards them and direct their behavior in socially appropriate ways. In the case of running around inside, that can usually be directed to outdoor play. But sometimes time restraints may mean you're unable to provide the alternative in the precise moment that you observe undesirable behavior. That's perfectly ok. You can provide it when both you and your child are calm and have some time that you can spend together.

Allow for Repetition

Children with ASD often feel an impulse to repeat activities. This is encouraged in the Montessori method, especially when your child wants to repeat a Montessori activity or a lesson. When repeating an activity, your child is strengthening connections and picking up new information. Much like the second or third time reading a novel allows you to discover nuances in the plot, repeating an activity allows for new discoveries.

Many children insist on reading the same book over and over, to the desperation of many parents who know the book by heart backwards and forwards. The familiarity of the text, however, allows children to pick up more difficult vocabulary words and learn the story. There's nothing wrong with reading it repeatedly, except that you might go crazy!

If you're concerned about your child excessively repeating an activity or book, try allowing your child to repeat, but with a slight variation. For example, when reading a book for the umpteenth time, try leaving out the last word of each sentence to see if your child can say it. Or, ask your child to tell you the story in the book while looking at the pictures.

Slight variations to Montessori activities are often available as extensions, or gradually more difficult tasks using the same material. If your child loves the Pink Tower, for example, have them set it up laying down instead of standing up. Then, have them set up the Brown Stair alongside it. Your child could also trace the base of each Pink Tower block, starting with the biggest, one inside the other. With these slight variations, you'll allow for repetition, but also encourage your child to use the material in new ways.

Guide to Useful Skills, but Don't Force

Following the child also involves encouraging independence by helping our children learn to do things on their own. Montessori believed that all children have a desire to become independent. From personal hygiene tasks to getting dressed and putting on shoes, gently pushing children to do things for themselves helps children on many levels. Even when your child doesn't initiate the desire to learn these skills, you can ask your child to try some steps on their own. Little by little, they'll learn to take care of themselves more and more. In addition to increased self-confidence and independence, these activities help develop both fine and gross motor skills.

Take Advantage of Interests

Many children, including children with ASD show a strong, specific interest. Whether it's a superhero, video game, favorite animal, color or other interest, you can use this as an opportunity to connect with your child. Follow their interest and dig deeper into it with them. Discover ways to learn through the lens of their interest.

If the interest is dinosaurs, make dinosaur art. Research the dimensions of dinosaur footprints, then make some together. Visit museums. Read books. Draw dinosaurs. Put together chicken bones into a model like paleontologists do with dinosaur bones. Learn dinosaur names. Design a dinosaur based on the different features they can have (horns, frills, quadrupedal or bipedal). The possibilities are endless, and this is true with any subject or interest. With a bit of creativity, we can help our children explore the subject of their passion in great detail covering a range of subject areas.

Seek Help

There's no doubt that you may run into times in your journey of following your child when you won't know what to do. When this happens, seek help. Find support from an educator, psychologist, therapist, online forum, friends and family. There are also many helpful community groups and autism research groups and foundations committed to helping families of children with ASD. By using the available resources and reaching out for support, you'll find new and better ways to meet your child's needs.

Prepare Your Spirit

One of Montessori's core beliefs was that teachers need to prepare themselves spiritually. As she states in *The Discovery of the Child*: "*She must acquire a moral alertness which has not hitherto been demanded by any other system, and this is revealed in her tranquility, patience, charity, and humility. Not words, but virtues, are her main qualifications.*" While it's impossible to be tranquil, patient, charitable and humble always (we're not super heroes!), this should be our goal. Avoid beating yourself up when you fail to follow your child perfectly or respond in the best way to a meltdown. Rather, be compassionate with yourself as well.

To reach these lofty goals, self-care is paramount. Make time for a 15-minute morning walk, an evening soak in the tub, a weekly fitness class, or another outlet. This time to yourself will give you a sense of peace and more patience for interacting with your child.

With your spirit cared for, you'll also be more likely to truly follow your child, have the patience necessary to understand their behavior and respond to it in the most constructive way. As some say "Happy parent, happy child." Or is it the other way around? Perhaps it works both ways.

"No one can be free if he is not independent..."
- DR. MARIA MONTESSORI

CHAPTER SEVEN

Managing Choice and Freedom

In my experience as a teacher, I found that many students came into the classroom knowing exactly what they wanted to work on. If there was a science experiment going on in the corner, many students would come in and check on that first. Others would head straight to the reading corner. In the preschool classroom, some students loved to see what the latest materials were on the practical life shelves. Nearly all of them loved beginning sewing lessons. Throughout the day, children move from one activity to the next in a series of decisions they make largely on their own. Students are invited to presentations with the teacher who carefully guides and orchestrates the activity in the classroom.

Choice and freedom in the classroom can be overwhelming for some students, hindering their productivity and ability to progress. This can happen for both neurotypical and children with ASD. What can we do to support choice and freedom at home and at school?

In this chapter, we'll discuss the importance of freedom and choice in Montessori, and also learn why this can be challenging for ASD students. Then, I'll offer some strategies for increasing your child's ability to manage freedom and choice.

Freedom and Choice in the Montessori Method

In our lives as adults, we make decisions constantly. It's an important survival skill. But, even many adults struggle with choices. For example, prioritizing a task list incorrectly can mean you need to stay up late to finish a project due at work the next day. Or, a struggle to choose what to purchase at the grocery store can reveal that we haven't prepared ahead of time with a meal plan or even taken a quick inventory of the pantry. These seemingly mundane skills all boil down to choices we make that can either enhance or add stress to our lives.

The Montessori method aims to prepare students to handle complex decision-making from the very beginning of their schooling. Beginning with choice in activities (as long as certain routines and rules such as cleaning up are being followed), students are slowly given more responsibility. In the elementary years, Montessori students are encouraged to organize and execute field trips to nearby attractions or community institutions. By middle school, they might plan a trip that lasts a few days and involves several hours of travel. At the heart of the method is the child's ability to move freely in the classroom, choose activities and progress in their learning in a self-directed way. The ultimate goal? Confident adults who are skilled at managing decisions in their lives from buying groceries to making career choices.

How does the freedom manifest itself exactly? Every Montessori classroom is unique. Yet, they all have the thread of freedom in common that's a function of the classroom setup and guidance from teachers. Shelves of materials, books and command cards are arranged according to subject area. After receiving a presentation, children are free to work with the material as they please, as long as another child isn't using it. Starting in elementary grades, lists, work plans or student-teacher meetings are sometimes used to help keep track of progress. But on a day to day basis, students enjoy a great amount of freedom in what work to do, where to do it and when.

This ability to handle freedom responsibly doesn't come automatically. Rules and routines are taught in the classroom so that students are aware of the expectations in the classroom. Using a rug or table for work, cleaning up each material after using it and placing it in the correct place when done are some of the basics. Students must also use a quiet voice in the classroom, avoid disturbing others and wait their turn to use materials that others are using. Only some materials and activities can be used or done in pairs or groups.

The Prepared Environment

Why did Montessori include this element in her classroom design? In addition to believing that freedom and choice are important life skills to learn how to handle, she also knew that allowing freedom in the classroom also goes hand in hand with following the child. You can't follow the child if they are completely restricted. Montessori carefully orchestrated the freedom and choices that children would have in the classroom.

She did this by building a prepared environment, the classroom, for the children she was working with. She made sure that there were plenty of interesting, engaging activities available that she knew would catch the children's attention. Distractions were kept to a minimum, with no loud, glitzy posters or excessive noise. Rather, the attention of the children was drawn towards the learning materials, which were the most exciting.

Guiding Towards Using Freedom and Choice Responsibly

Children with ASD are often particularly sensitive to routines. It can be very upsetting for a child with ASD to make changes from a routine. In the Montessori setting, a child with ASD might grow accustomed to selecting the same material to work with at the beginning of work time. If another child chooses the material before them, it may ruin their whole morning. Under these circumstances, it might seem impossible for the child to choose another material and have a productive work time.

For this and other reasons, freedom and choice can be challenging for children with ASD to manage. While other children may revel in the opportunity to choose, this may even feel like a burden for some children with ASD. However, there are ways that children can learn to handle the responsibility and overwhelming aspects that choice and freedom present.

First, let's consider some of the models offered by examples of children with ASD in Montessori schools. Michelle Lane for example, shared that in her school, there was a range of choice that occurred. With children most severely affected by ASD, one-on-one teachers were provided. Most Montessori materials were provided in the classroom, but it was the teacher who guided and directed the use of the materials, rather than the child. As children increased in their abilities, or with children who require less support, teachers worked with up to two students at a time. In the Lane Montessori School for Autism setting, you can see that freedom and choice don't play as large a role in the classroom as is typical in the Montessori setting. This is in response to the greater need for guidance.

Another experience, shared by Lois Omonde, shows a different way of approaching routines and freedom for a child with ASD who is part of a larger Montessori classroom. In this setting, there are many more distractions and options to choose from. After all, the environment has been created for an entire classroom full of different needs, rather than how in Lane's school, classrooms were small, for just one or two students. In this setting, Omonde says, a designated desk was provided for the child in a quieter area of the classroom. Freedom of movement was limited to encourage concentration, which as discussed, is one of the first keys for success.

Omonde also mentioned that she created a visual chart for the student so that he could follow a daily routine. The upper elementary-aged child was expected to complete activities in math, reading and language daily. In addition, computer time could be earned by finishing required works.

However, there was a great deal of freedom afforded. Omonde says they accessed many books to support learning and followed the student's interests in trains, spiders, animals and Harry Potter. It's also important to note that the boy had an IEP, and although he had access to and used the Upper Elementary curriculum, he moved at his own pace.

Other Montessori experts and teachers have also commented on the possibility of using the method with ASD children. Some common themes are an encouragement for high functioning ASD students to be integrated into Montessori classrooms. While most Montessori schools don't offer a combined ABA/Montessori teaching methodology, many Montessori teachers also speak positively of also including lower functioning ASD students in the classroom with the assistance of an aide or one-on-one teacher accompanying them.

An aide can provide the support and guidance that children with ASD need in an environment that, although calm and conducive to learning, may be challenging due to the choice and freedom afforded. In a typical Montessori classroom, neurotypical children may also struggle to handle freedom responsibly. Within the method, there's a strong theme of "freedom within limits," which children must master. When children struggle with this, Montessori teachers often guide by gently limiting freedoms and providing greater direction for the child. For example, a new child in a preschool classroom may be limited to using items from certain shelves, or even be asked to pick between two materials to use. As the child shows greater responsibility, greater freedoms are afforded.

What are some practical ways to help guide choice and freedom?

Create Structure with a Chart

Keeping in mind that every child is unique and will have a different reaction towards choice and freedom, similar strategies to those described above can be used. When a child arrives as a newcomer to a Montessori program, it's not uncommon to limit choices. Having the child use items from a certain shelf or providing additional guidance and support when picking materials is quite normal. For children with ASD, this approach is a good start, but working out a routine and representing that visually is often the most helpful. For pre-literate or non-verbal children, images or pictures of the materials that will be used can be printed to create the schedule. These sorts of supports can be very helpful for adapting to this new way of doing things.

In addition, some children may benefit from additional structure. For example, Lois Omonde noted that she and her student often used a silent timer to encourage him to complete tasks. I also noticed the difference between two students on the ASD spectrum during my time teaching in the lower elementary classroom. While one student struggled to finish tasks, another finished them without any external intervention at all. The first student, however, was highly motivated by creating a checklist of the work he wanted to complete and then crossing off each activity as he finished it.

It's likely that there will be a different, unique, solution for each child with autism. All children are unique and what motivates them, makes them tick and makes learning enjoyable is different for each child.

Slowly Offer Choice

Over time, you can slowly offer the child some choice in the activities. First, you might offer that the child changes the order of the routine. Or, you may consider offering two new materials, and have the child choose which one to try that day. In this way, the child slowly takes more control over their learning.

Why offer choice if things are going well with structure and support? Externally imposed structure requires constant reliance on an adult, or outside force to regulate what's going on. To achieve true independence, children must be able to make decisions and make use of freedoms, not just in the classroom, but in life. By starting out in a safe, controlled environment and slowly shifting the responsibility of choices to the child, greater independence is achieved.

Observe

Make sure you keep observing the child to ensure that needs are being met. For example, in addition to a daily schedule, you may discover that a weekly schedule should also be posted somewhere in the room for the child to see. Or, perhaps you'll learn that the child is very motivated in some academic areas and can be allowed greater choice within certain subject areas. Most importantly, the child should be viewed as the main indicator of what's working well, or not so well. Changing several items in a routine at once could be stressful for one child, but could mean improvements for another. With careful observation, you can help guide a shift to greater independence and freedom.

Allow Observing

One important element of a Montessori classroom is the opportunity children have to observe one another. Children are free to observe another child working, as long as they are respectful and don't interfere. Montessori believed that this was a strong motivating factor, especially for the younger students in the mixed-age classroom. Many students with autism, as well as neurotypical children benefit greatly from observing. In addition to Montessori's insights on observing in the classroom, a wealth of autism experts and organizations agree that allowing students to observe before being asked to try something can be very helpful. Lois Omonde shared, "What worked for my student was I would model what he should do. Then, he would practice until he could do it." The organization, *Montessori Education for Autism*, also agrees, arguing that some students with autism may engage in "third party participation", observing other students use a material many times. Even if the child never decides to use the material on their own, they can benefit from this interaction.

While limits on observing should be imposed when children interrupt or distract others, this is also a skill that can be worked on and learned. Children with autism can become unobtrusive observers and gain much from the ability to stand-by and watch others when participating is too difficult.

Over time, with guidance, most children can gain greater independence and make more and more choices in the classroom or with regards to their education. By empowering children to make decisions with regards to their education, their agency can be increased.

"The consciousness of knowing how to make oneself useful, how to help mankind in many ways, fills the soul with noble confidence, almost religious dignity."
- DR. MARIA MONTESSORI

CHAPTER EIGHT

Grace and Courtesy Lessons and Children with ASD

"Today, we're going to practice answering the phone," said my co-teacher during circle time. The children's eyes lit up as she pulled out an old phone from behind her. The children eagerly took turns picking up the phone saying "Hello. This is..." filling in with their name. David, a student with ASD also gave it a try.

He was often shy around new people and just a bit awkward at times. Whenever someone new would come in, he would often hide behind one of his teachers. However, in these moments of practicing social skills, he was often able to imitate what others were doing.

Children with ASD struggle with even the most basic social skills such as looking someone in the eye and recognizing emotions in others. In the Montessori curriculum, children learn social skills explicitly and are guided towards being self-reflective individuals who are respectful and kind to others.

This aspect of the Montessori method is beneficial over several levels for children with ASD. For inclusive Montessori classrooms where children with ASD are part of the community, the grace and courtesy lessons help ensure that the classroom is a welcoming space for all students. On another level, the explicit highlighting of social skills can help students with ASD understand social norms they might otherwise never notice.

Montessori included this area in the curriculum because she believed that education was not just for academic purposes, but to help prepare children's spirits. She had much greater expectations for education than what are traditionally named. An advocate of peace, Montessori is famous for saying *"...establishing lasting peace is the work of education; all politics can do is keep us out of war."* This quote comes out of Montessori's strong belief in shaping children to become peaceful individuals who work together, are respectful and who know how to live in community. To this end, she included education of the spirit in her curriculum, in a specific series of lessons.

Examples of Lessons in Grace and Courtesy

You can work with your child on some of these lessons to enhance their ability to interact with others.

Emotional Awareness

For many children with ASD, recognizing emotions in others can be challenging. In this lesson, children can work on identifying different emotions. Print out photos of people making different facial expressions representing different emotions. These should be photos of real people, not emojis or illustrated images. Start with the simplest ones such as sad, happy and angry.

To start, see if your child can identify each of the emotions. If not, conduct a 3-period lesson to teach the names of each emotion (reference the explanation of the 3-period lesson in chapter 4 if necessary). If possible, ask your child to imitate each of the faces during the first period. This can be tough for children with ASD, but it's a skill that can be developed. Point out specific areas of the face such as the mouth and eyes, and how they change with each emotion.

You can then use these cards in many other activities. Throughout the day, you might ask your child how they're feeling and why. You can get out the cards so that your child can pick which one they identify with at the moment.

Another helpful activity is during reading time. While reading a picture book, identify any feelings the characters feel and match it to the card. It's also important to discuss why the characters may feel this way. This is a skill developed in neurotypical and children with ASD alike. Children are usually unable to imagine that someone else might have a different perspective or have different feelings than them until after the preoperational stage which lasts from about age 2-6, according to Piaget. Although children can see when someone else is crying and understand that they're upset, it can be hard for them to identify why. By talking about how other people (or book characters) feel, we can help children grasp this concept, which is vital for interpersonal relations.

Basic Social Skills

Many basic social skills may seem every day and ordinary to us, but are a bit strange for children. By making a lesson out of it, you can help provide context for your child. Here are just some of the social skills that you can teach:

- How to introduce yourself
- Saying hello
- Shaking hands
- Saying goodbye
- Introducing someone else
- Asking to join a group/play
- Inviting someone else to join a group/play
- Saying "Thank you"
- Saying "excuse me"

- Asking for help
- Apologizing

Each of these lessons focus on teaching the skill, role-playing and discussing the context in which the skill is used. Just because you teach these sorts of lessons won't mean that your child will automatically start using them spontaneously on their own. Lots of encouragement, practice and support is needed. Rather than forcing your child to use these skills in real-life, wait until it happens naturally, providing support and practice along the way.

As you'll notice, most of the lessons here relate to manners and relating to others in a socially acceptable way. For children with autism, this can be a life-changing opportunity to learn how to interact with others. As adults, we also begin to recognize just how many social skills may not be obvious to our children.

I've been in this situation many times with my own children. Take interrupting for example. How do children interrupt? Often, they yell or come up to us and just start talking, even if we're in the middle of a conversation. If I found myself sighing in exasperation as my four-year-old interrupted me as I was speaking with my husband about something we had to sort out. I had probably just scolded him for doing it, and yet here he was again. On comes our reptilian parent brain that throws logic out the window and we often find ourselves wanting to just shut our kids up (just for one minute!) Yet, I realized that I had never actually bothered to teach him how to interrupt. "That could be a learned skill," I remember thinking to myself. Yes, perhaps we all learn it eventually by simple observation, but there's no reason I couldn't talk to him about it and ask him to change his behavior. And what do you know, he got it! We practiced him walking in and saying "excuse me," in a pleasant voice while standing next to us patiently. He got what he needed, our attention for a minute, and we could then move on with our conversation.

Of course, it doesn't stick automatically. We must continue practicing. And it may take some time for you to achieve your goal with your child, but it is possible. It does require that we change our approach, though, and remember to demonstrate each skill that we'd like to see our children use.

Peace

Montessori included themes of peace throughout her curriculum for students of all ages. Starting with the youngest of students, conflict resolution is taught using the peace corner, which is also a place where students can go to center themselves when feeling upset, sad or angry. You could even say that this element of the classroom takes student's mental health into account, encouraging the expression of emotions in a safe space rather than expecting students to charge on and continue working.

The elementary Montessori curriculum focuses on peace in a special way. Montessori noticed that children become much more interested in social interactions around the age of 6 or 7 and this lasts throughout the early elementary years. To capitalize on this interest, Montessori encouraged students to work together in the lower elementary classroom and also included a special peace and cosmic education curriculum for students in this age group.

The peace corner at the elementary stage grows in complexity. Now, rather than only focusing on self-reflection and solving interpersonal conflicts, the peace curriculum includes four areas of focus: self-awareness, community-awareness, cultural awareness and environmental awareness. Children are invited to be peaceful in all of these areas. In self-awareness, this may mean naming one's own emotions and taking time for self-care. Community-awareness refers to being peaceful with friends, family, classmates and others we meet in life. Children are encouraged to show kindness through actions and words in the community. Cultural awareness means learning about and respecting the great diversity that exists in the world and living together peacefully. Finally, environmental awareness refers to our responsibility to acknowledge the effects of our actions on the environment. When discussing this area, students may develop actions plans for their lives and at school to live in harmony with the environment.

This sort of curriculum can enrich your child's emotional and social life. Through the four different areas of the peace curriculum, children gain a greater appreciation and understanding of each human's role in the world.

Although your child may not become a social butterfly because of these sorts of lessons, they can certainly go a long way in helping your child feel more comfortable during social interactions. Sometimes having a predictable script to start out with can relieve anxiety and diminish the unknown in social interactions. What's more is these lessons can help cultivate independence, which is one of the main goals of the Montessori method.

"Respect all the reasonable forms of activity in which the child engages and try to understand them."
- DR. MARIA MONTESSORI

CHAPTER NINE

Understanding and Responding to Triggers for Children with ASD

Within minutes of walking into the classroom, Brian was crying. It seemed like the challenge of working in the classroom was overwhelming for him. Sometimes he would crawl under a table or chair, curl up and wail and wail. When talking with his behavioral therapist, she suggested that we let him cry, not remove him from the situation and encourage him to take part in classroom activities. If we didn't insist on it, she said, he would never get used to school.

Unfortunately, in his family, there was very little structure and Brian was used to getting what he wanted. This had resulted in him refusing to participate at school sometimes. Although at times, he could waltz into the room, pick up the sound cylinders and get right to work, other days he would go straight into melt-down mode.

Many children with ASD experience triggers. While the example above focuses on a child being pushed slightly outside of his comfort zone, there are many different types of triggers that can affect children. For each child, it might be something different. I knew a young man with autism for example who always needed to wear a hat. Although he learned to take it off at school, he always put it back on as soon as he went outside. I distinctly remember a moment when he was asked to take off his hat outdoors to be able to see the conductor (he was playing bells on the sideline in the marching band). He ended up getting very upset about it.

Other children, like Lois Omonde's student, don't like loud noises. Fire drills were too much for him, so Omonde, would take him on a walk before the drill so that he didn't hear the loud bell so close by. In addition, he didn't like when other people touched him or gave him hugs.

Chances are you've noticed some triggers that are affecting your child as well. But, why does this happen?

Understanding Triggers

Children with autism experience, sense and perceive things differently than we do. When you hear a door slam, it might sound like thunder to your child. Or you slip on a cozy wool sweater, but to your child it may feel like a metal brush or a thousand mosquito bites. Although you enjoy the different textures that food has, your child might experience it like eating stones and so seeks out smooth applesauce, yogurt and pudding.

Just like for you, a variety of experiences and events may lead you to feel a certain way, the same is true for your child. However, the difference is that things that seem normal to you, such as turning on the lights, may be just as stressful for your child as it is for you to get a lecture from your boss.

The first step in understanding triggers and their subsequent behavioral consequences is accepting that your child experiences things differently than you do. As has been discussed earlier, sensory integration is a common difficulty in children with ASD. Your child may easily become overwhelmed with an excessive amount of visual stimuli, touch or noises. In addition, the sense that controls balance, the vestibular system, and proprioception, which is the sense of one's body in space, both contribute to feeling overwhelmed. When the sensory information isn't processed correctly, the meltdowns and other behavioral outcomes such as becoming withdrawn, screaming, crying, kicking or engaging in self-stimulatory behaviors result.

There are many different types of triggers. While many are sensory-related triggers, there are also other types, or combinations of factors that can result in a meltdown. It can be helpful as a parent or teacher to know ahead of time what may affect a child with ASD. This way, you can be emotionally prepared for the child's impending behavioral response, help develop coping mechanisms, and sometimes avoid the triggers altogether.

Tracking Your Child's Triggers

It can be hard sometimes to pinpoint what exactly is causing your child's outbursts and meltdowns. In fact, sometimes you won't be able to at all, and that's ok. However, by observing patterns, you can begin to discover some triggers that may be affecting your child.

Start by getting a notebook or creating a document to track your child's behavior. Note down even mundane things about the time or day that your child has an outburst. For example, you may write down what they had to eat, what time of day it was or if it was raining, etc. You may begin to notice patterns regarding your child's behavior and eventually pinpoint some of the triggers that are affecting your child.

Through this tracking exercise, you may also discover what makes your child's life easier or more enjoyable. Keeping an open mind to what may be affecting your child is key. Remember that your child experiences the world in a different way than you do.

Dr. Martha Herbert and Karen Weinstraub discuss some helpful areas to consider when tracking triggers, which include:

The senses

As has been discussed, sensory experiences and a distinct way of processing sensory stimuli can create an overwhelming situation for a child with ASD, resulting in a meltdown.

Social situations

Children with ASD often struggle to interpret social situations. Body language and social signals such as someone showing boredom or other emotions can be like a foreign language to them. Yet, this doesn't mean that children with ASD never notice if others are making fun of them or that they don't need friends. Some children with ASD may feel left out, while others happily wander around at recess on their own. You may discover that social situations can put your child in a bad mood or result in them feeling withdrawn or experience difficulty concentrating afterwards. If your child goes to school and experiences difficulties after recess, for example, the social aspect of this time in the day may have played a role.

Communication struggles

Especially if your child has limited verbal abilities, communication struggles can be a trigger. Imagine if you couldn't express yourself or communicate your wants, needs or thoughts to anyone else? It would most certainly be frustrating at times. Even if your child is verbal, there are times when children can be experiencing something, but be unable to talk about it. Strong feelings or emotions can overwhelm their ability to communicate.

Boredom (lack of stimulation)

Montessori believed children want to be engaged in work. Interesting work. Any child, including children with ASD, may exhibit poor behavior due to something as simple as boredom. While it's important for children to find their own ways to deal with boredom, it's also our responsibility as adults to ensure that the necessary tools and activities are accessible so that children can engage in stimulating work. When engaging work isn't possible, coping mechanisms can also be taught. Is your child in a boring environment? A long car-ride, time waiting at the doctor's office, or a lesson in a not-so-favorite subject at school can result in your child expressing their boredom through their behavior.

Pain

Especially for children who are non-verbal, it may be difficult to know if a child is experiencing pain. A sore in the mouth, stomachache or headache could be affecting your child. Children who are on the verge of getting sick may exhibit grouchier behavior than usual or may have more meltdowns as well. Try to look for signs such as your child curling up in a ball, rubbing their stomach or pulling at their mouth as indicators of pain.

Food allergies or sensitivities

It's been known for some time now that people may be affected in different ways by certain foods. Lactose intolerance, for example, can result in discomfort in the stomach, putting your child in a bad mood. However, other food items and additives such as colorants, etc. have also been shown to have a strong effect on some individuals, changing their behavior. Sugar is another contributor. You can keep a food journal or use an elimination diet to help determine if your child has any food allergies. Consulting with a specialist can also help ensure that you're taking all of the necessary steps to discover food allergies and sensitivities.

Hunger, thirst, feeling tired

Who doesn't feel a bit grumpy when they're hungry, thirsty or tired? Following Maslow's hierarchy of needs theory, when these most basic needs in life aren't met, it's nearly impossible for energy to be focused on other needs such as friendship, meaningful work and more. So, you're likely to see more outbursts and negative behaviors after a poor night's sleep or when your child is hungry or thirsty.

Emotional environment

Whether children are aware of what's going on, it's easy for them to soak up the emotional environment around them. If there's an environment filled with stress at home or school, your child is likely absorbing it. Feelings are contagious. Whatever the dominant mood is where your child spends time, they will probably pick it up, which might result in undesired behaviors.

Coordination struggles

All young children must gain fine and gross motor skills through practice over time. Because of deficiencies in the vestibular (balance) and proprioception (special awareness) systems, children with ASD may struggle even more with coordination. This can be extremely frustrating. Imagine knowing what you want your body to do, but being unable to execute it. A lack of control over the body often results in an expression of frustration, stress or anxiety, especially when the stakes are high. For example, gym class, when other children are observing physical performance, can cause anxiety before and after the class.

Routine Changes

This is another common trigger for children with ASD. Doing anything out of order, even something as simple as brushing teeth after breakfast instead of before-hand, can result in a meltdown. Larger changes such as field trips, vacations and other events can cause extreme stress and worry for children with ASD.

Avoiding and Coping with Triggers

Now that we have a greater understanding of what triggers may affect your child, what should you do once you know what they are? The best response to triggers is two-pronged. In some circumstances, you may want to remove triggers from your child's life. But, it's also necessary to recognize that eliminating all triggers isn't a solution that is helpful in the real-world. Triggers will appear in the real-world, whether you'd like them to or not. As part of developing independence and being able to participate fully in life, children with ASD need to experience life as it is, which sometimes involves triggers. Here's where the second approach, which is teaching and developing coping skills, comes in.

With some triggers like food allergies or sensitivities, it's clearly preferable to avoid them altogether. Other triggers like being overwhelmed with sensory input are likely something that your child will encounter in life over and over again. There are many products and techniques that you can use to help your child cope with overstimulation. For example, many people with autism make use of sound-canceling headphones to reduce background noise that can be overwhelming.

Other coping techniques may include practicing breathing slowly, closing one's eyes for a few minutes, or taking a "sensory break." This last popular and effective option has even been implemented in some schools, according to *Edutopia*. Using sensory rooms, children can meet their sensory needs which has a calming effect. These rooms may include items like a padded floor or cushion for laying on and crashing into, exercise balls for bouncing on, swings, a light wall, and more. Depending on the space you have available, you might consider creating a sensory space for your child where they can meet sensory needs, especially when feeling out of sorts.

For routine changes, it's wise to let your child know ahead of time that there will be a change. This will help your child be prepared for what might happen. Consider going through uncomfortable situations they may encounter as a result of the change. For example, if your child is going on a field trip, talk about going on the bus, noisy, excited kids, etc. Then, detail ways that your child can cope with these changes. For example, remind your child they can put their sound-cancelling headphones on (if relevant) or that they can ask a teacher to go to a quiet place for a break.

Jaco, a boy with autism was made famous when his father, Richard Mylan, created a documentary about their life. Jaco takes a video of his experiences as a coping mechanism. His father remarked that later, they look through the videos again together, and it provides a way for Jaco to process events in his life. Jaco's videos about his visit to BBC are now quite famous and easily found on social media.

This example shows us that coping mechanisms can be unique and creative. If possible, work with your child to discover the options together. For example, ask "what can we do if things get too loud all of the sudden?" You may be surprised by your child's response. In this case, you might brainstorm a few ideas such as: ask others to be quiet, use music, use sound-canceling headphones, close eyes and take a deep breath, use ear-plugs, etc.

With regards to basic needs like sleeping, eating and drinking, teaching your child good habits is the best place to start. Choose a reasonable bedtime and enforce it so that your child won't be excessively tired during the day. Offer your child healthy food options and keep water handy throughout the day. The Montessori method encourages children to be involved in cooking and food preparation. Make sure your child has access to healthy snacks and water throughout the day and provide lessons for how they can prepare things to eat on their own. You may consider using a low cabinet to keep plates and healthy snacks that your child can access. This will help them independently manage these basic needs.

Within the Montessori method, the environment and curriculum are supportive of students with ASD because many triggers are avoided and healthy coping mechanisms are taught. This helps create a space that's conducive to learning for children with autism. Below, I'll outline some of the ways that the Montessori environment helps avoid triggers and supports coping mechanisms.

The Montessori Environment and Curriculum and Triggers

There are many things unique to the Montessori method that make it an ideal space for children with ASD. Here are some of the ways the Montessori environment and curriculum help:

The Classroom

The good news is that a Montessori environment is usually much more calm and quiet than traditional classrooms. The Montessori environment includes few distractions in decorations and posters on the wall, but typically features neutral tones and a few decorative items.

The focus within the classroom are the learning materials displayed in wooden boxes, baskets and on trays.

Children are expected to work quietly throughout work time, which usually lasts for about 3 hours at a time. There are some materials and presentations in the classroom that involve noise, but generally the classroom is quiet.

These factors are helpful for children with autism because visual and auditory stimulation are low, meaning that distractions are few. Because children are free to move about the classroom, some areas are busier than others. Teachers can guide children with ASD to quieter areas to work with fewer distractions.

Snacks and Water Available

The triggers of hunger and thirst are avoided in the Montessori classroom. Children are usually allowed to snack or get a drink of water whenever they choose to do so.

Social skills support

As was discussed in the previous chapter, the Montessori curriculum includes a robust section of grace and courtesy lessons. Here, social skills are highlighted and taught to children. Rather assuming that all children know how to say "hello," for example, even this most basic skill is taught, often in a group lessons. Recognizing emotions, sharing, introducing oneself, introducing others, and many other lessons that advance in skills and difficulty are included in the curriculum. What's more is lessons about being kind to others, inviting others to play and similar inclusion-oriented lessons are taught, making the classroom a welcoming space for all students. These sorts of lessons can be especially helpful for children with autism who may not naturally observe and imitate social courtesies and norms. By breaking down each skill into pieces, the child can learn how to do it, and when.

Coordination work

In the Montessori curriculum, both fine and gross motor skills are practiced. Specific activities, especially in the infants and primary programs (covering ages 0-6), were developed by Montessori to help children improve their coordination. Activities that focus on coordination are used throughout the curriculum, but the bulk can be found in the practical life and sensorial areas. Gross motor skills are practiced within the classroom when moving furniture, but activities such as walking around the circle and others are also included.

Over time, practice with coordination can improve performance, reducing frustration, stress and anxiety that the child may experience.

Emotional – Peace Corner

The classroom is generally peaceful and provides a positive emotional environment for children. However, Montessori recognized that children may bring a range of emotions with them to school, and experience others while there. The Peace Corner is an important area in the classroom, that can be used at all levels although the bulk of the available curriculum surrounding this area is at the elementary level. What is the Peace Corner exactly? It's a comforting space where children who are feeling sad, angry or upset can go take a break. Children who have gotten into an argument can also use this space to resolve their conflicts.

A Peace Corner can also be adapted to a home situation. Typically, the Peace Corner is a small, out of the way space filled with pillows. A few comforting images or works of art can be included. Then, depending on the preferences of the child, a mini Zen garden can be used, an hour glass, some flowers, a fountain, some stress balls or stacking rocks can be added to give children a peaceful activity to do in the space. Children are invited to use the space whenever they need it. You can suggest this as a space your child may want to use when they become frustrated or anxious about something.

Communication through materials

For children who have low verbal skills, the Montessori method provides relief from all of the talking. Most materials in the infant and primary program focus on using the hands and working with materials. The presentations are focused on the materials and aren't very language-heavy most of the time. When there is a lot of language, there are always visual representations for children to see.

The language area of Montessori provides a simple way to build vocabulary. One common activity is to label the classroom. Another popular material for beginning reading, the pink material, includes single-word cards that are matched with images. These can be used to help build vocabulary as well as support beginning reading.

Because the method is personalized for each student, it's also easy to incorporate language support systems such as keyboards or PECS (Picture Exchange Communication System). Depending on what system you use with your child, this can be incorporated into your Montessori homeschooling routine or you can discuss it with your child's teachers.

Responding to Outbursts the Montessori Way

Inevitably, there will be times when your child responds strongly to a trigger or not getting what they want. Melt-downs, crying, outbursts, screaming, aggression and other responses are common and are normal responses to feelings of stress, frustration and overwhelm. These are challenging behaviors for parents and teachers to respond to. The Montessori method offers some insights into how to respond during these difficult times.

As a doctor, Montessori strived to meet all of her patient's needs. Some report that she was just as likely to recommend that a family make chicken soup as she was to prescribe medicine. With a holistic approach to the person, and in understanding triggers for children with ASD, our response to outbursts should be in part to help meet needs.

However, in the heat of the moment, it's unlikely your child is open to taking a sensory break, going to the peace corner or using another helpful coping mechanism. Here are some helpful steps that can help you handle your child's outbursts:

1. **Identify Trigger**

    While your child is crying or lashing out, try to identify what may have triggered your child and what they are trying to communicate. If you are unable to do so, remember to mark it down in your trigger notebook so that you may be able to understand it later.

2. **Change Spaces**

   Whether you can pinpoint the reason for your child's behavior or not, try to get to a safe space where your child can complete their outburst. If you're out shopping, for example, try to get to the car or a park where things are a little less tense and there aren't so many people around.

3. **Name it**

   If you know why your child is upset, try naming it for your child. For example, "I see you're angry we couldn't find your favorite crackers at the store. That would make me upset too." Or, "There's too much noise here. I know that bothers you." By naming what's going on, you'll help your child improve their ability to self-regulate and identify when they need to make use of healthy coping mechanisms.

4. **Keep Limits You've Set**

   If your child is upset because you've said "no" to something, stick to it. Don't give in to your child just because a storm is brewing and you can see an outburst is coming. For any child, limits are very important. If you've decided that TV time is over or that your child can't have one more cookie, don't turn around on your decision. This is inconsistent and will only confuse your child more, as well as encourage tantrums and outbursts. In any discipline situation, your "no" should be "no," just like your "yes" should be "yes."

5. **Get Sensory**

   When your child has an outburst, depending on your child's unique personality, you may be able to begin a sensory break to help them calm down. For example, if your child likes to bounce on an exercise ball, bring the ball in and invite them to do that. Or, massage your child's back if this would be comforting. With young children, you may find that just holding them close or swinging them back and forth can help them calm down. As you observe your child's self-stimulatory behaviors and notice what sensory experiences they seek out most, you can discover what may also work in crisis situations.

6. **Stay Close**

   Otherwise, you can calmly wait beside your child until the outburst has run its course. During the outburst, you can remind your child, "I'm right here with you. I'm sorry you're feeling so bad." At home, you can just check-in regularly throughout the outburst so that your child knows that you're close by for support. This communicates to your child that feelings are ok.

7. **Safety First**

   If at any point your child tries to hurt themselves or others, intervene. Setting these firm limits that tell your child that they cannot harm others is important. Physically restrain your child, or if this is impossible or unsafe, remove the other child or individual from the situation. You can say something simple, like "You may not bite" or "I won't let you hit me."

Keep it short, no need to get into long, confusing explanations. Your child isn't ready to listen or discuss at the moment. You need to just be clear, and keep everyone as safe as possible.

8. **Don't Shush**

    It's important for parents to let children know that expressing these emotions, even if extreme, is ok. By trying to get your child to stop or be quiet will only allow the tension and stress to continue building up. Try not to take outbursts personally. They are an expression of strong feelings and nothing else.

When It's Over

When you're both calm again, you can go over what happened and practice some coping mechanisms for a situation similar to what happened. Autism expert Christine Reeve suggests doing a "social autopsy" on some socially related struggles. The steps outlined in this process can be helpful for dissecting just about any situation that results in an upset. Here are some of the steps. I've modified to make them fit in better with the Montessori philosophy:

1. What happened? Try talking through what happened, especially the cause of the outburst or upset. Help identify feelings, especially if others were involved. Be matter of fact. For example, "You were angry and wanted the ball. Dan wanted the ball too." Children with autism may not be able to recognize that their friend also wanted the ball. By reviewing, you can help them understand better what happened.
2. Note reactions. For example, "You pushed your friend" or "You screamed." Dr. Reeve calls this step "identify the mistake." Her intention is to have the child identify the behavior

that should be changed. However, I think it's just as easy to avoid using this word, and simply talk about reactions and expressions of emotion. For example, "You were angry and so you screamed. It's ok to be angry."
3. Identify who was affected. This is important. Try to notice how both the child and others were affected by the behavior. For example, "Dan was hurt when you pushed him." Or, "You cried for a long time and missed arts and crafts."
4. Find solutions. Encouraging apologies to those who were affected is great. However, remember that children also have their own way of making up, and forcing an apology won't make it genuine. The ultimate goal should be to cultivate empathy, understand the consequences of the actions and be positive about the future. Solutions for the future may include practicing a new coping mechanism ideal for the situation that occurred. Other options include reviewing already known coping mechanisms, journaling about the event, drawing a picture about using a coping mechanism, etc.

Keep in mind that you don't need to dissect every single situation your child runs into. These in-depth reviews can be helpful for the most explosive or severe situations. Another key point to make this process successful is that you don't completely relive the situation all over again. The idea isn't to rehash what happened, upsetting your child and rubbing in their struggle. If it doesn't feel helpful in the moment or your child gets upset, stop. You can always try again later.

As with any response to behaviors, try to be predictable and consistent. Especially for children with autism, it can be very confusing if you respond to them calmly one day and yell the next. Maintaining consistency will help your child learn to make changes in their behavior and choose to use appropriate coping mechanisms when presented with difficult situations and triggers.

Try to be creative with your solutions. If your child responds to a frustrating social situation by hitting, one option could be to punch pillows or a punching bag. Or, if your child runs away when they get upset, you could allow the running, but decide with your child where they're going first or ask if you can run along. This way, you're allowing their natural coping mechanism to run its course, but also keeping your child safe.

Finally, there are situations unique to each child and family that may require professional support. Talk to specialists about any behavior issue that you can't seem to find a solution for. A professional, outside opinion can often go a long way in finding a new, creative way to deal with the problem.

CHAPTER TEN

Conclusion

The Montessori method can be a wonderful way to help guide children with autism, respecting their unique needs, perspectives and interests while also encouraging their independence and growth. This holistic philosophy addresses all areas of life, giving parents and educators support in how they should react to behaviors and interests and how to approach everything from academics to practical life skills and social skills. Children with autism, just like all children, have amazing potential. The Montessori method allows the possibilities to be unlocked and explored fully.

With the new vision of children's inner life that Montessori provides, you can work more harmoniously with your child on achieving goals. Rather than fighting against interests, you can follow your child and use them as a vehicle for learning. Lessons can help develop social skills, improve response to sensory stimuli and build vocabulary. With independence as a main goal and carefully guided principles that respect the unique characteristics of every child, Montessori is the perfect match for children with autism.

What's next? Depending on how you've decided to include Montessori in your child's life, you can take additional steps to learn more about the method. If you are planning to homeschool, you can either piece together or purchase your own curriculum. There are many resources available in the form of books and online blogs that can help you learn more about the method and take on homeschooling. On the last few pages of the book you'll find a list of helpful resources you can access. I highly recommend digging into Montessori's own writings. Although they can be a challenging, intense read, there's much to be gained from reading her ideas directly.

I encourage you to get started by really taking the main principles of Montessori's philosophy to heart. Following your child, their pace, interests and trying to understand their behavior are the most important first steps towards beginning to use the method. Your reaction to your child's behaviors using the method is also an important area that can produce a positive change in your relationship with your child. Slowly, you can begin to incorporate early intervention activities and sensorial, social skills and other lessons into your lives. However, the preparation and spirit of the educator, Montessori tells us, is vital to successfully implementing her philosophy.

Although you may feel overwhelmed and that there's a lot of work for you to do, take things one step at a time. You don't have to begin all at once. Plan out one change or one lesson to try each day. As you grow in your knowledge, understanding and comfort with the method, you can incorporate more and more.

I wish you the best on your journey in Montessori with your child.

More Titles by Rachel Peachey

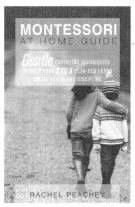

Montessori at Home Guide: Gentle Parenting Techniques to Help Your 2 to 6-Year-Old Learn Social Skills and Discipline

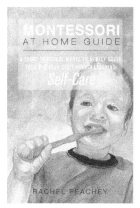

Montessori at Home Guide: A Short Practical Model to Gently Guide Your 2 to 6-Year-Old Through Learning Self-Care

More Titles by the Producers, A. M. Sterling

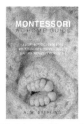

Montessori at Home Guide: A Short Introduction to Maria Montessori and a Practical Guide to Apply Her Inspiration at Home for Children Ages 0-2

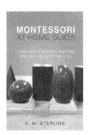

Montessori at Home Guide: A Short Guide to a Practical Montessori Homeschool for Children Ages 2-6

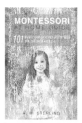

Montessori at Home Guide: 101 Montessori Inspired Activities for Children Ages 2-6

Resources

www.montessori.org
www.montessoriforeveryone.com
www.montessorieducationforautism.com
www.montessoriautism.com
www.autismspeaks.org
www.autism.com
www.autismclassroomresources.com

References

2016, Online. "Sensory Activities For Children With Autism". *Ldalearning.com*. N.p., 2017. Web. 7 June 2017.

"ABA: Behavioral Treatment | Autism Research Institute". *Autism.com*. N.p., 2017. Web. 7 June 2017.

"Autism And GI Disorders". *Autism Speaks*. N.p., 2017. Web. 7 June 2017.

"Autism's Associated Medical Conditions". *Autism Speaks*. N.p., 2017. Web. 7 June 2017.

"Autism Behavior Problems: What's Triggering Your Child's Outbursts?". *Helpguide.org*. N.p., 2017. Web. 7 June 2017.

"B.F. Skinner's Behavioural Theory". *Kidsdevelopment.co.uk*. N.p., 2017. Web. 7 June 2017.

"BBC Autism Challenging Behaviour". *YouTube*. N.p., 2017. Web. 7 June 2017.

"Biography Of Dr Maria Montessori | Association Montessori Internationale". *Ami-global.org*. N.p., 2017. Web. 7 June 2017.

Bourne, Lori. "An Interview With Michelle Lane Of The Lane Montessori School For Autism". *Montessoriforeveryone.com*. N.p., 2017. Web. 7 June 2017.

"CDC Update On Autism Shows Gap Between Early Concerns And Evaluation". *Autism Speaks*. N.p., 2017. Web. 7 June 2017.

"Challenging Behaviors Tool Kit". *Autism Speaks*. N.p., 2017. Web. 7 June 2017.

Christensen, Deborah L. et al. "Prevalence And Characteristics Of Autism Spectrum Disorder Among 4-Year-Old Children In The Autism And Developmental Disabilities Monitoring Network". N.p., 2017. Print.

DeVita-Raeburn, Elizabeth. "Is The Most Common Therapy For Autism Cruel?". *The Atlantic*. N.p., 2017. Web. 7 June 2017.

"DISCUSSION PAPER: Maria Montessori". *Swaraj.org*. N.p., 2017. Web. 7 June 2017.

Dvorsky, George. "Why B.F. Skinner May Have Been The Most Dangerous Psychologist Ever". *Io9.gizmodo.com*. N.p., 2017. Web. 7 June 2017.

"Facts About Asds". *CDC - Facts about Autism Spectrum Disorders - NCBDDD*. N.p., 2017. Web. 7 June 2017.

"Facts About Asds". *CDC - Facts about Autism Spectrum Disorders - NCBDDD*. N.p., 2017. Web. 7 June 2017.

"Floortime". *Autism Speaks*. N.p., 2017. Web. 7 June 2017.

Friedman, Amanda Joy. "Answers: Beliefs About ABA". *Psychology Today*. N.p., 2017. Web. 7 June 2017.

"Genius Locus". *The Economist.* N.p., 2017. Web. 7 June 2017.

Haelle, Tara. "Majority Of Autism Increase Due To Diagnostic Changes, Finds New Study". *Forbes.com.* N.p., 2017. Web. 7 June 2017.

Irinyi, Michelle. "Autism And Special Needs Children In The Montessori Classroom". *Montessoritraining.blogspot.com.* N.p., 2017. Web. 7 June 2017.

"Jacob And His Piano". *Autism Speaks.* N.p., 2017. Web. 7 June 2017.

Janes, Robyn. "Autism In Early Childhood Education Montessori Environments: Parents And Teachers Perspectives". *Aut.researchgateway.ac.nz.* N.p., 2017. Web. 7 June 2017.

Lane-Barmapov, K. Michelle. "Montessori And Autism: An Interpretive Description Study". (2016): n. pag. Print.

Lantz, Johanna. "Play Time: An Examination Of Play Intervention Strategies For Children With Autism Spectrum Disorders". *Iidc.indiana.edu.* N.p., 2017. Web. 7 June 2017.

Margolis, Amy, and Michael P. Milham. "44.0 Neural Circuitry Underlying Three Common And Often Co-Occurring Childhood Disorders: Autism Spectrum Disorder, Attention-Deficit/Hyperactivity Disorder, And Learning Disorder". N.p., 2017. Print.

Marshall, Chloe. "Autism And Montessori". N.p., 2017. Web. 7 June 2017.

Mazumdar, Soumya et al. "Spatial Clusters Of Autism Births And Diagnoses Point To Contextual Drivers Of Increased Prevalence". N.p., 2017. Web. 7 June 2017.

"Montessori And The Child With Special Needs - Montessori For Everyone - Montessori Blog". *Montessori for Everyone - Montessori Blog*. N.p., 2017. Web. 7 June 2017.

"Montessori History | Grand Forks Montessori Academy". *Grandforks-montessori.com*. N.p., 2017. Web. 7 June 2017.

Montessori, Maria, and Mary Anderson Johnstone. *The Discovery Of The Child*. 1st ed. Delhi: Aakar Books, 2013. Print.

Montessori, Maria, Anne E George, and Henry W Holmes. *The Montessori Method*. Print.

Montessori, Maria. *The Absorbent Mind*. Print.

"New Government Survey Pegs Autism Prevalence At 1 In 45". *Autism Speaks*. N.p., 2017. Web. 7 June 2017.

"New Study Of Autism Prevalence In 4-Year-Olds Underscores Need For Earlier Detection". *Autism Speaks*. N.p., 2017. Web. 7 June 2017.

"Research: Autistic Savants | Autism Research Institute". *Autism.com*. N.p., 2017. Web. 7 June 2017.

Park, Elizabeth. "A Mixed Methods Case Study Of Montessori Pedagogy For A High-Functioning Autistic Child". *Academia.edu*. N.p., 2017. Web. 7 June 2017.

Reed, Sheri. "My Autism Story: The Boy Who Feels No Pain". *CafeMom*. N.p., 2017. Web. 7 June 2017.

Reeve, Christine. "Autism Classroom Resources - Where Research Meets The Classroom". *Autism Classroom Resources*. N.p., 2017. Web. 7 June 2017.

"Richard & Jaco: Life With Autism - BBC Stories". *YouTube*. N.p., 2017. Web. 7 June 2017.

"Richardandjacobbcbreakfast". *YouTube*. N.p., 2017. Web. 7 June 2017.

Rogers, Sally J., and Geraldine Dawson. "Early Start Denver Model For Young Children With Autism". *Google Books*. N.p., 2017. Web. 7 June 2017.

Schopler, Eric, and Gary B. Mesibov. "Learning And Cognition In Autism". *Google Books*. N.p., 2017. Web. 7 June 2017.

"Self-Stimulatory Behavior | Autism Research Institute". *Autism.com*. N.p., 2017. Web. 7 June 2017.

"Sensory Integration | Autism Research Institute". *Autism.com*. N.p., 2017. Web. 7 June 2017.

Solomon, Andrew. "The Autism Rights Movement". *New York Magazine*. N.p., 2008. Web. 7 June 2017.

"Stephen Wiltshire". *En.wikipedia.org*. N.p., 2017. Web. 7 June 2017.

"Supporting Learning In The Student With Autism". *Autism Speaks*. N.p., 2017. Web. 7 June 2017.

"The Montessori Method.". *Digital.library.upenn.edu*. N.p., 2017. Web. 7 June 2017.

"The Sensory Room: Helping Students With Autism Focus And Learn". *Edutopia*. N.p., 2017. Web. 7 June 2017.

"What Does The Word 'Autism' Mean?". *WebMD*. N.p., 2017. Web. 7 June 2017.

"What Is Autism? - Autism Society". *Autism Society*. N.p., 2017. Web. 7 June 2017.

Zeliadt, Nicholette. "Early Therapy May Seed Lasting Gains In Children With Autism | Spectrum | Autism Research News". *Spectrum | Autism Research News.* N.p., 2017. Web. 7 June 2017.

About the Author

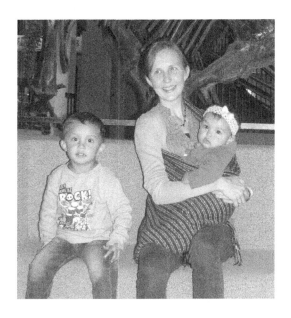

Rachel Peachey is a Montessori teacher, freelance writer and mom of two little ones. She enjoys living in beautiful Guatemala with her husband and children who were born in 2013 and 2015. She devotes her free time to homeschooling her kids and running a community library she began in 2016 at the local Catholic church.

Visit her website and blog: http://www.rachelpeachey.com/

About the Publisher

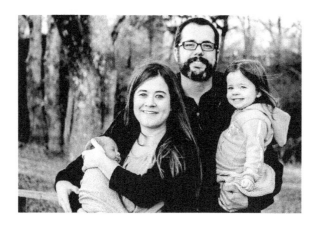

Ashley and Mitchell Sterling are new author/indie-publishers and video-bloggers on YouTube known as 'Fly by Family'. When they're not writing, or talking to a camera lens, the Sterlings value their time together, in beautiful eastern Kentucky, where they live with their two children, Nova and Mars.

Visit their website: http://www.sterlingproduction.com/
Visit them on YouTube: http://www.youtube.com/flybyfamily

Thank you for reading this *Sterling Family Production* book! We would love to hear from you in an honest review on Amazon! Reviews help the author and us to improve what we do, as well as to get to know you, our readers.

Sincerely,
Ashley and Mitchell Sterling

Made in United States
North Haven, CT
24 February 2023